Contents

Foreword   vii
Acknowledgements   ix

1   What is Asthma?   1
Need to breathe   2
Lung structure   2
The airway tubes   4
Mucus clearing   7
Airway inflammation   8
The muscle layer of the bronchioles   8
Bronchial 'twitchiness'   9
Reversible and non-reversible airways obstruction   10
Definition of asthma   11
Diagnosing asthma   11
Who gets asthma?   12
International differences   13
Recent trends   14

2   Diagnosing Asthma   15
Symptoms   16
Physical examination   16
'Lung function' tests   17
Patterns of peak flow readings   21
Response to treatment   23
Limitations of PEFR readings   23
Chest X-rays   24
Blood and 'allergy' tests   25
Antigens and antibodies   25
Asthma and allergy   26
Difficulties in diagnosis   30
Severity of asthma   33

3 The Causes of Asthma   35
Cells of the immune system   35
Risk factors for asthma   37
Host factors   37
Environmental factors   39

4 Treating Asthma (1) – Minimising Trigger Factors   47
Identify trigger factors   48
Identify atopy   49
Stop smoking   50
House dust mite   51
Animals   54
Moulds   54
Pollens   55
Exercise   56
Drug therapy   56
Food allergy   56
Desensitisation   57

5 Treating Asthma (2) – Drug Therapy   59
Steroids   59
Sodium cromoglicate and nedocromil   61
Leukotriene receptor antagonists   62
Bronchodilators   62
Theophylline   63
Anticholinergics   63
Controllers and relievers   64
Antihistamines   65
Inhaler devices   65

6 Managing Asthma – Stepwise Treatment   73
Step 1   75
Step 2   75
Step 3   75
Step 4   76
Stepping down   76
Severe asthma   76
Anaphylaxis   78

7   Asthma in Children   80

8   Chronic Obstructive Pulmonary Disease (COPD)   82
Diagnosis   83
Treatment   83
Oxygen therapy   84
Surgery   85

9   Complementary Treatments for Asthma   86
Acupuncture   87
Homoeopathy   88
Exclusion diets   88
Other nutritional approaches   88
Breathing techniques   89
Hypnosis   89
Relaxation techniques   89
Chiropractic   90
Herbal medicine   90
Massage   91
Conclusion   91

10 Asthma in Special Circumstances   92
Pregnancy   92
Operations and anaesthetics   93
Asthma and sport   94
Asthma medication and sport   95
Scuba diving   95
Mountaineering and skiing   96
Finally   97

Appendix A: References   98
Appendix B: Drug Therapy: Class Examples   103
Appendix C: Useful Contacts   117

Foreword

Asthma, which is derived from the Greek word meaning 'to pant for breath', is a very common disease in the western world and in the last 20 years the number of people affected by it has more than doubled. Effective treatments are available which, although they are not curative, provide the asthma sufferer with good relief and control of their symptoms. Doctors and nurses are now well trained in diagnosing asthma as early as possible and in instituting appropriate treatment. The treatment of asthma should be regarded as a partnership between the patient and the doctor or nurse, and it is now agreed that the part played by the asthma sufferer in taking control of their own disease contributes to achieving a better outcome. This means that patients need to know as much as possible about this condition.

This book is aimed as asthma sufferers and their relatives – those who need to understand the causes and treatment of this common condition. It covers most aspects of asthma and provides very clear and up-to-date information in lay terms, including current reseaerch in asthma from which newer treatments may come.

To the asthma sufferer, the most important parts of the book include practical information about how to avoid asthma triggers, about tests that can be used to diagnose asthma, about how treatments work and how they should be correctly used, and about asthma under special circumstances (such as during pregnancy). Finally, advice is provided as to how the asthma sufferer can help themselves to control their symptoms.

The success of asthma treatments depends on the judicious and correct use of available medication, the adherence to prescribed treatments and the partnership between the medical carer and the asthma sufferer. This book will serve towards this purpose. I am sure that the asthmatic patient and the general public will find this book both informative and helpful.

Professor Kian Fan Chung MD DSc FRCP
Professor of Respiratory Medicine,
National Heart and Lung Institute, Imperial College London
and Honorary Consultant Physician,
Royal Brompton and Harefield NHS Trust, London

Acknowledgements

I am delighted to acknowledge the help of one of the world's leading asthma researchers, Professor Kian Fan Chung of the National Heart and Lung Institute, Imperial College School of Medicine, who kindly reviewed the information presented here despite many other commitments. He and the other members of the small army of people around the globe who work to understand this important illness deserve the thanks of all of us for making it an increasingly treatable one.

I sincerely thank Sarah Grant and Judith Longman at Hodder & Stoughton for their help and support in ensuring that this book became a reality, and Amanda Williams for making sense of my sketches.

Great care is taken to ensure that the NetDoctor Help Yourself to Health book series is as accurate and as up-to-date as possible and the responsibility for any errors is mine. Please let me know if you spot any or have any suggestions for improvement in this or any other book in the series. I can be contacted at d.rutherford@netdoctor.co.uk

Dr Dan Rutherford
Medical Director
www.netdoctor.co.uk

Chapter 1

What is Asthma?

No one definition of asthma completely describes it in all its aspects, but basically it is the condition in which there is reversible narrowing of the airway tubes of the lungs. Narrow tubes offer more resistance to the flow of air, so someone who has asthma may experience symptoms such as breathlessness, wheezing or cough. These are the common symptoms but two individuals with asthma do not necessarily experience asthma in exactly the same way. Among the differences between them for example are the 'trigger factors' that can set off an asthma attack. Therefore, to understand asthma more fully and to appreciate how the treatment for it works this simple definition needs to be expanded. Some background information on the lungs and how they work will make this much clearer, so for the moment we'll leave this 'narrow tubes' concept standing and make a digression into the structure of the lungs and airways.

Need to breathe

All living creatures, whether animal or plant and including the humblest bacteria, require a supply of energy to power the processes of life. Plants can trap energy from sunlight but animals are dependent on extracting energy from their food, via the myriad chemical reactions that occur within the body. Some microbes can successfully manage without oxygen (the brewing industry depends upon them entirely!) but in higher forms of life energy is released by the combination of oxygen with fuel. This process is called oxidation, and it produces waste products in the form of carbon dioxide and water. The main function of the lungs is to supply a means of taking in oxygen and of removing carbon dioxide. (The lungs also have important secondary functions. For example they are the site of action of enzymes involved in the general control of blood pressure, but these are not directly relevant to asthma and so are not considered further here.)

Lung structure

The lungs are made up of millions of tiny 'bubbles', called alveoli. Each single alveolus is like a miniature balloon made of an extremely thin membrane and connected at its neck to a tiny air tube, that links back, through ever larger tubes, to the main tube (bronchus) of each lung. The two main bronchi join in the centre of the chest to form the windpipe (trachea) that originates at the 'voice box' (larynx) in the throat. This is illustrated in figure 1.

Through the act of breathing each alveolus is alternately partially emptied and then re-charged with air. On the outside surface of the alveolus is a mesh of very small blood vessels called capillaries. These link the blood vessels carrying oxygen-poor blood from the body (pumped to the lung by the heart) to the blood vessels returning from the lungs to the heart, ready to be pumped out to the rest of the body. During their passage through these capillaries the red cells of the blood pick up oxygen from the air inside each alveolus. This is possible because the alveolar membrane is so thin that it poses little barrier to the passage of oxygen molecules across it.

Figure 1 (a): Main structure of trachea and bronchi

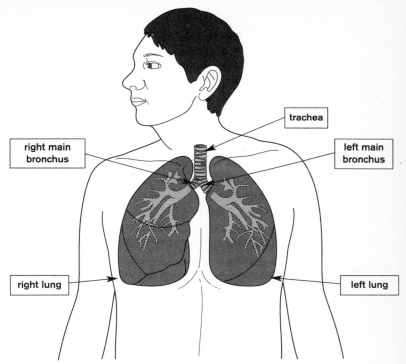

Figure 1 (b): Fine structure of alveoli

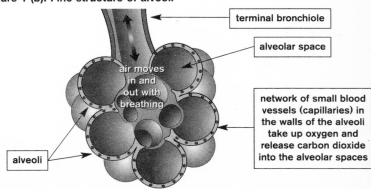

Carbon dioxide, the waste product of energy release by oxidation, is gathered by the blood that flows through every part of the body. In its journey through the alveoli carbon dioxide passes in the opposite direction to oxygen and enters the air space of the alveolus. From there it is breathed out. Thus blood is continuously re-charged with oxygen and stripped of carbon dioxide as it flows through the lungs.

The size of each alveolus is very small – about four times the width of a human hair – but there are approximately 300 million alveoli in a pair of lungs, so the total surface area of lung tissue involved in the process of gas exchange is very large.

It's important to realise that the 'business parts' of the lungs are the alveoli – they are the site of exchange of oxygen and carbon dioxide between blood and air. It is the job of the airway tubes, however, to deliver the air to each and every alveolus and it is within these tubes that the process of asthma exists. Asthma does not directly affect the alveoli other than to impede the delivery of air to them.

The airway tubes

Understanding asthma, and how to treat it, therefore requires more detailed knowledge of the airway tubes. First, the terminology:

TRACHEA
The trachea is the main windpipe. It starts below the larynx, the area below the base of the tongue where the vocal cords are situated, and goes down the middle of the front of the throat. Deep within the middle of the chest (about the level of the middle part of the breast bone) it divides into the bronchi – one to the right lung and one to the left.

BRONCHI
The first divisions of the trachea are more exactly known as the right main bronchus and the left main bronchus. Thereafter each main bronchus divides repeatedly into smaller and smaller branches (bronchi) to reach all areas of each lung – the term 'bronchial tree' is very apt.

The walls of the trachea and the bronchi contain rings of cartilage – a springy, tough material that gives the tubes strength and flexibility and keeps them open. You can feel these rings in your own trachea if you gently run your fingers across its surface just below the 'Adam's apple'. Between the cartilage rings the walls are made of muscle.

BRONCHIOLES

By the time each bronchus has divided about six to eight times the width of each branch is just a few millimetres across and a change takes place in the structure of the walls. Cartilage disappears and muscle becomes predominant. The bronchioles divide further until the smallest type, called the 'terminal bronchioles', are formed. Each terminal bronchiole is connected to a small group of alveoli (see figure 1). Often doctors refer to 'large' and 'small' airways, meaning the trachea/main bronchi and smaller bronchi/bronchioles respectively.

Detailed structure of the bronchioles

Figure 2 shows the structures you'd see if you looked down a high-powered microscope at a healthy bronchiole cut across the middle. The bronchiole is quite open, with a relatively wide channel for air to pass. Lining the bronchiole is a thin layer of cells that have various different roles. Some produce mucus, which coats the lining cells and traps any particles that are inhaled. Other cells are members of the immune system, on the lookout for foreign invaders such as bacteria and viruses. Others are structural support cells. Within the wall of the bronchiole is a thin layer of muscle.

Compare this with a bronchiole from someone with asthma, as represented in figure 3. Here the inner layer of cells is thicker, due mainly to infiltration by cells from the immune system. Mucus-producing glands are more numerous and produce plugs of mucus that lie in the airway channel, partially blocking it. Some of the lining cells are shed and lie as clumps mixed with the mucus, adding to this blockage. The muscle layer and surrounding support tissues are much thicker and the result is a much narrower air channel. This combination of several changes in the structure of the airways in asthmatic people

Figure 2: Cross section of normal bronchiole

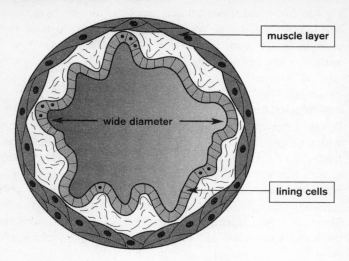

muscle layer

wide diameter

lining cells

Figure 3: Cross section of bronchiole in asthma

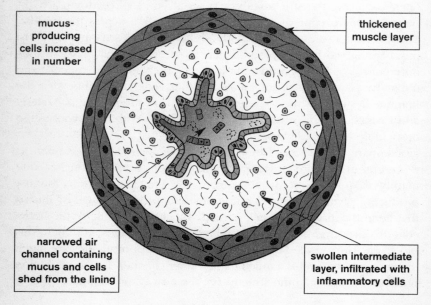

mucus-producing cells increased in number

thickened muscle layer

narrowed air channel containing mucus and cells shed from the lining

swollen intermediate layer, infiltrated with inflammatory cells

is called 'airway remodelling'. It occurs throughout the bronchial tree but has its greatest impact in the small to medium-sized airways where constriction has its main effect upon airflow.

Coughing is a reflex that can be triggered by many factors but in asthma it occurs in response to an awareness that the bronchi are partially blocked. First the vocal cords are closed together, preventing the escape of air from the lungs. Then contraction of the chest wall muscles and the diaphragm builds up air pressure within the chest. Opening the vocal cords suddenly releases this pressure at high speed, which helps blow open any blocked air tubes as well as propel mucus higher up the bronchial tree where it can eventually be cleared away.

Mucus clearing

Mucus is a very important part of the lung's defence against infection or other form of attack by dust, pollen, pollutants and all the other particles we breathe in every day. However, simply producing mucus does not solve any problems unless there is a system for getting rid of it. As is so often the case, Nature's solution to this problem is ingenious. Microscopically small hairs cover the exposed surfaces of the cells that line the entire bronchial tree, as far down as the terminal bronchioles. These tiny hairs, called cilia, beat continuously in an upward direction, constantly nudging the mucus along towards the larger bronchi. Ultimately this mucus stream is either swallowed or spat out. Cilia also cover the lining of the nose and sinuses and work in the same way to keep these areas clean. In healthy people the incessant mucus 'circulation' goes more or less unnoticed but when something like a chest infection comes along the extra mucus produced becomes all too obvious.

One of the many ill effects that are caused by smoking is paralysis of the cilia. Once they stop beating mucus plugs build up, hence the characteristic need for smokers to continuously cough up the mucus that they can't clear properly. The intense irritation of tobacco smoke stimulates more mucus glands to develop, so producing more mucus, which of course adds to the problem.

Increased mucus production is also seen in asthma, probably as a reaction to the inflammation within the bronchi, which is the basic process that drives asthma along. Sticky thick mucus is much harder for the cilia to move, and it will be obvious that the combination of smoking and asthma is a particularly bad one.

Airway inflammation

In medical language the term 'inflammation' is really a shorthand way of saying that the immune system is involved, usually to an excessive degree. The immune system is complex and has multiple parts, but among the most important are populations of specialised cells in every part of the body that are tuned to recognise the presence of foreign material or organisms. These monitoring cells can themselves act to destroy the invaders but more importantly are able to send out chemical signals to recruit more cells from the immune system to come and help. Generally these arrive via the bloodstream but in longer lasting inflammatory situations the immune system cells replicate locally and can build up to a considerable degree. This is a characteristic finding in asthma, as was seen in figure 3, where the infiltration of the inflammatory cells caused the bronchiole lining to be much thicker than normal. As will be seen in later chapters, strategies to reduce this inflammation or prevent it occurring are among the central methods of treating asthma. Much of the research into asthma is concentrated on the behaviour of the immune system in the lungs.

The muscle layer of the bronchioles

The bronchi and bronchioles are not just passive tubes conducting air in and out of the alveoli – they are much more active than that. In particular the presence of the muscle layer in the bronchioles means that their diameter can vary, depending on the state of contraction or relaxation of the muscle. The muscles are arranged in spiral fashion around the walls, so that when they contract the airways become narrower. When the muscles relax then the airways open up. Over-activity of the muscle layer, causing constriction of the tubes, is another major aspect of asthma.

SMOOTH MUSCLE

There are two main types of muscle in the human body, described according to their general appearance when looked at by microscope. Striped (or 'striated') muscle is the type that generally moves under our voluntary command. It is therefore the type of muscle we have in our limbs, fingers, chest wall, abdomen, scalp – in fact anywhere there is a muscle that we can move at will. Striated muscles contract or relax according to the commands sent to them by the brain through the nervous system. This isn't a complete description of striated muscle – for example the heart is made of a variety of striated muscle yet it is not under direct voluntary command – however it is a good enough classification in general terms.

Smooth muscle is the type that lines the bronchial tree as well as all of the blood vessels throughout the body, the lining of the digestive system, the bladder and the womb. Like striated muscle, smooth muscle responds to signals from the nervous system but this is largely from the 'automatic' part of the nervous system, i.e. the part that is *not* under voluntary control. The other main influence on the activity of smooth muscle is the presence of hormones, either produced locally by specialised cells in the adjacent tissues or carried by the bloodstream from a hormone-producing gland elsewhere in the body. Usually a combination of nervous and hormonal control applies to each smooth muscle tissue. There are subtle differences between the smooth muscles in different parts of the body, which make them sensitive to different hormones.

The medical term used for the degree of activity or tension within a muscle is its 'tone'. Factors that alter the tone of the muscles within the bronchi therefore have great relevance to asthma.

Bronchial 'twitchiness'

The medical jargon term for this property is 'hyperresponsiveness' and it means the tendency seen in asthma for the airways to close up with much less provocation than is the case in people who don't have asthma. One can do this in the laboratory by getting people to inhale substances known to make airway muscles go into spasm (bronchoconstrictors) and then measuring how 'tight' their tubes appear to be. In asthma a smaller dose of the irritant will cause more marked and longer lasting airway blockage than in someone who is not asthmatic. Outside of the laboratory this hyper-responsiveness shows up in practical terms as the symptoms of asthma (breathlessness, wheeze, cough) that can be brought on by inhaling an irritant like tobacco smoke, by an abrupt change in air quality, by catching an airway infection or even following exercise.

Reversible and non-reversible airways obstruction

The ability of the smooth muscle of the bronchial tree to both relax and contract means that the degree of airway obstruction can vary – sometimes very widely. When an asthmatic person is in a good spell, perhaps because of effective treatment or because they have not been exposed to anything that can trigger the asthma for a while, then they may have little or no obstruction present. If they then come into contact with a triggering agent to which they are particularly sensitive then they might experience symptoms of asthma quite quickly – sometimes in only a few minutes – although usually asthma will get worse over days or even weeks. Some asthma treatments are very quick acting, so the symptoms might just as quickly be relieved by, for example, the right sort of inhaler.

In asthma the characteristic aspect of the airways obstruction is that it is *reversible*, at least to some extent. Later in the book some other lung conditions will be covered that also cause airway blockage but which have little or no degree of reversibility. These are not asthma, although it is true to say that this distinction is not always clear. In other words there are many conditions that can cause airways constriction, the commonest of which is asthma, but in asthma the constriction is reversible to a greater or lesser degree.

As we saw earlier, some of the narrowing of the airways that occurs in asthma is due to the changes that occur in the numbers and types of cells that build up as well as the thickening of the muscle layer and other tissues – the 'airway remodelling' process. This is not so easy to reverse, and perhaps in all people with asthma one has to say that although treatment can markedly reduce the amount of airway inflammation it can't remove it altogether. Asthma can therefore be treated but we can't claim yet that it can be cured.

Definition of asthma

Bringing together the points raised in this chapter and adding some other known facts allows a more precise definition of asthma to be made:

- Asthma is a common inflammatory condition of the airways, whose cause is not completely understood.
- As a result of the inflammation the airways are hyper-responsive and they narrow easily in response to a wide range of trigger factors.
- This causes symptoms such as coughing, wheezing, chest tightness and shortness of breath. These symptoms are often worse at night.
- Airway narrowing is usually reversible but in some people with longstanding asthma the inflammation may cause a degree of irreversible airway obstruction.

Diagnosing asthma

A complete definition also includes details of the characteristic findings one can see down a microscope in the lung tissue of someone with asthma but clearly that is no practical help in day-to-day life. It is technically feasible to safely take a piece of lung tissue for analysis and in some lung diseases this is necessary in order to make a complete diagnosis, but not usually for asthma. A doctor makes a diagnosis of asthma based mainly on the history of the typical symptoms along with findings on examination of the patient. Sometimes it is obvious that asthma is present but quite often it is not. Being told that you have asthma is an important event in someone's life, so the issue of making an accurate diagnosis is covered in more detail in the next chapter.

It is important to emphasise that asthma is a 'clinical diagnosis', i.e. it is the combination of the 'symptoms and signs' rather than laboratory tests that define whether someone has asthma. There is no blood test, scan or X-ray that can say for sure that you do or do not have the condition. There are ways of trying to confirm the presence of asthma (which are dealt with in chapter 2) but it is worth remembering that there can be differences between countries and even between individual doctors in how asthma is detected and diagnosed.

Who gets asthma?

Asthma can affect any individual at any age and is one of the commonest medical conditions world wide. It is commonest in early childhood – as many as 30 per cent of infants in the UK have been wheezy in the first year of life. About a third of children up to the age of three have asthma symptoms but two thirds of these children will be symptom-free by the age of six. In a large survey of schoolchildren in the UK aged 12–14 (part of the 'ISAAC' study – International Study of Asthma and Allergies in Childhood – see appendix A) one in five had been diagnosed with asthma at some point previously. In Western countries asthma is now the commonest reason for a child to be admitted to hospital.

CHILDREN
The main factor responsible for wheeze appearing in very young children is virus infection of the airways – something that all children are prone to get as they come into contact with the world around them. Most of these children are not asthmatic. As children get a bit older and reach primary school age then allergy, rather than infection, is the most common underlying reason for them to wheeze. Those children who show a tendency from infancy to also be allergic (for example if they also have the itchy, dry skin condition called eczema) are more likely to keep getting attacks of wheeze as they get older and therefore to become 'properly' asthmatic. Between 10 and 20 per cent of children with asthma carry it with them into adulthood. The factors associated with those who are most likely to do so are dealt with in chapter 3.

Statistics are interesting when taking a broad view of asthma in the population, but they don't help much in predicting whether any particular child who is wheezy when young will 'grow out of it' as he or she gets older. Most of the time one just has to wait and see what happens, and treat the wheeze as necessary in the meantime. In fact it may be doubtful whether people who have asthma in childhood really do ever leave it completely behind them. It is difficult to put an exact figure on it but a significant proportion of adults who seemed to have lost their earlier tendency to be asthmatic will get obvious asthma again in adulthood or will show a hidden tendency for asthma when subjected to tests of their lung function.

ADULTS

Asthma can develop for the first time in adulthood. Sometimes this is because of occupational exposure to agents that can cause asthma or which bring it to the surface in someone who has an underlying tendency to the condition. Adult-onset asthma can also develop without any recognisable exposure or other known cause. There is no upper age limit for the development of asthma – it has developed for the first time in people in their nineties. Asthma is probably under-recognised in the elderly because there are so many other conditions that cause similar symptoms and therefore mask its presence. There is therefore little accurate information about how common asthma is among the oldest section of the population but between 10 and 23 per cent of adults in Britain up to about 60 years old have either been diagnosed with asthma or give a history of recurrent wheeze over the preceding 12 months.

International differences

The ISAAC study showed striking differences between countries in the percentage of schoolchildren who reported asthma-type symptoms over the preceding year. Unfortunately, with a score of 30 per cent, the UK tops the league. New Zealand, Australia, Republic of Ireland and Canada are the other members of the top five. The countries where the symptoms were least commonly reported included India, China, Eastern Europe and the former Soviet Union. There is insufficient information to say if these differences stem from variations in the environment, industrialisation or other factors that can trigger allergic conditions.

Recent trends

One of the biggest concerns about asthma is that it is getting commoner, at least in the affluent countries where it is already a major problem. Although heightened public and medical awareness of asthma means that it is now better recognised and therefore more commonly diagnosed, this does not account for most of the upward trend. Two to three times as many children are now being diagnosed with the condition compared to about twenty years ago, yet it remains unclear which are the most important factors driving this change.

Certainly it appears that urban dwelling and higher material standards of living are associated with a greater tendency for children to have asthma compared with developing countries. But when one looks at which groups *within* affluent countries are the most likely to get asthma then one sees higher rates among low-income and minority group families. Inner-city dwellers are worse off, in part because they are more likely to have damp, poorly ventilated houses and to be more exposed to environmental attack from traffic pollution and the like. Of course these are generalisations – asthma is still common among children from more prosperous and better-housed sections of the population. There are a great many complex interacting forces involved in determining who will and who won't develop asthma and we are a long way from knowing what they all are.

SUMMARY
- Asthma is a longstanding inflammatory disorder of the airways.
- Airway inflammation causes restriction of airflow through them. In asthma this is mainly reversible but it can become irreversible.
- The main symptoms of asthma are breathlessness, wheeze and cough.
- Asthma can affect all age groups but is commonest in childhood.
- Asthma affects people from all countries but is commonest in affluent Western populations.
- Asthma is becoming commoner.

Chapter 2

Diagnosing Asthma

Asthma is a treatable condition, but it is not a minor one. Being diagnosed with asthma is therefore a significant event and it is important that the diagnosis is correct. There are many possible reasons why someone may cough, wheeze or become breathless and asthma is only one of them. Conversely, it is not necessary to have all these symptoms for asthma to be present. Children especially may just have a persistent cough for example.

In making a correct diagnosis in the full medical sense a doctor has to eliminate all the other conditions that could share the typical symptoms of asthma, but to go through all of these here would be far more likely to confuse than clarify the issue. It is more helpful to cover the patterns of symptoms that are suggestive of asthma, along with some of the methods that can be used to confirm the diagnosis on those occasions when it is unclear.

Symptoms

Several more specific symptoms are highly suggestive of asthma. The following list is from a questionnaire developed by the International Union Against Tuberculosis and Lung Disease that has often been used in surveys to reliably detect people with asthma.

Have you at any time:

- had wheezing or whistling in your chest?
- had an attack of shortness of breath that came on following strenuous activity?
- had an attack of shortness of breath that came on at rest during the day?
- woken up with an attack of wheezing or ·coughing?

A positive response to any of these questions is suggestive of asthma and if you have replied 'yes' to them all then it is virtually certain you are asthmatic.

Other clues to asthma that become more obvious with the passage of time are:

- Colds that always 'go to the chest' or take more than 10 days to improve.
- The presence of wheeze, chest tightness or cough after exposure to certain trigger factors (e.g. animal fur, pollen).

It used to be said that 'not all that wheezes is asthma', but asthma is now so common that it is probably more accurate to say that 'all that wheezes is asthma until proven otherwise'.

Physical examination

When a doctor makes a physical examination of a patient he or she is looking for the presence of extra clues that will help make a diagnosis or will directly or indirectly help in the assessment of a particular aspect of a person's health. The value of physical examination varies a great deal depending on the nature of the condition that is being assessed. In skin disease, for example, the visual appearance of a rash may be all that is needed to diagnose it precisely. In asthma, however, the amount of information a doctor may gather from examination can vary between nil (i.e. there are no abnormal findings) to a cluster of signs that make it obvious that asthma is present.

When someone has a particularly bad attack of asthma the muscles of the rib cage and of the diaphragm have to work extra hard to overcome the resistance of the narrow bronchi to the movement of air. Sometimes this can be seen on inspection of the chest as a movement of the muscles between the ribs. This is usually apparent only in thin people or in children. Someone who shows this 'physical sign' is usually struggling for breath. Fortunately most attacks of asthma are nothing like bad enough for this to happen, and the doctor's inspection of the chest will usually not reveal any abnormality.

Listening with a stethoscope to the chest can, however, reveal noises that point to the presence of asthma. A stethoscope is a very simple device that merely transmits the vibrations on the surface of the chest up to the ears of the doctor or nurse via tubes. Prior to the invention of the stethoscope the doctor simply pressed his ear against the skin of the patient. The stethoscope is more efficient as it gathers sound over a wider area and then funnels it into the tubes, effectively amplifying the sound. In someone with an asthma attack the typical sounds are of a musical whistling noise, most obvious on breathing out. There may also be crackles heard if there is a lot of mucus lying in the tubes. When someone has a particularly bad attack of asthma they may be unable to get much air in and out of their chest, and in those circumstances there can paradoxically be very little wheeze to be heard.

The presence of a wheeze over both lungs is strongly suggestive of asthma but the reverse is not true, i.e. it is perfectly possible to have asthma and have a completely clear chest when sounded by the stethoscope. The basic nature of the airway narrowing in asthma is that it is variable and therefore can be difficult to confirm.

'Lung function' tests

Medical textbooks on the detailed measurement of airflow in and out of the lungs look complicated enough to deter most people other than specialists in chest medicine. Coping with asthma on a day-to-day basis you do not need to know a lot about tests of lung function (a fact that most doctors who aren't chest specialists are happy about too!). However, one common measurement that is helpful to understand is the 'peak expiratory flow rate', usually abbreviated to 'PEFR' or 'peak flow'.

The PEFR is simply the maximum speed at which a person is able to blow air out of their lungs and the principle behind it is quite straightforward. If you have ever tried to empty the air from a bicycle pump while holding your thumb over the exit hole you will already know that the smaller the hole the harder it is to force out the air. Similarly, if the bronchi are narrowed then it is harder for the muscles of the chest to shift air in and out of the lungs. At any point in time the maximum speed at which someone can empty their lungs of air therefore depends to a large extent on whether their bronchi are narrowed or open. Of course a large fit adult will be able to exhale more air more quickly than a child (and men tend to have higher peak flow readings than women) but by making corrections for age, sex and build one can say whether a person is at or below the PEFR one would expect. There are charts and ready reckoners that allow this to be done easily and the GP or practice nurse will do this initially so that an asthmatic person knows what is average for their age and height, etc. A low PEFR therefore suggests narrow bronchi.

Even more helpful is the fact that by following the pattern of the peak flow readings over days or weeks one can get extra information that helps assess how well controlled an individual's asthma actually is. For example, if an asthmatic person catches a cold and notes that their peak flow falls over the ensuing few days then they will know to increase their asthma treatment to try to prevent it becoming any worse. Peak flow readings are measurable, so they can put a figure against how 'tight in the chest' someone feels. Some people with asthma find that they show a change in their peak flow reading before they notice much alteration in their symptoms. For them the peak flow reading gives an early warning of worsening of their asthma, allowing them to make adjustments to their treatment in good time and thus minimise the amount of trouble they get.

Simple 'peak flow meters' are available on prescription. Low reading meters are suitable for children and for adults with severe lung impairment – these give more accurate results at the lower end of the scale. Children younger than five or six are not really able to use peak flow meters very well, and to ensure that they don't get confused between breathing out for the peak flow meter and breathing in with their inhaled medicine it's best not to use these meters until they are a bit older.

The commonest design of meter is tube shaped and inside the tube is a snugly fitting slider that can move freely when air is blown into the mouthpiece of the device. Attached to the slider is a marker that runs in a slot on the tube casing, on which is a scale marked off in 'litres per minute' (L/min) – the units of measurement of peak flow. The faster the puff of air that someone can blow out then the higher up the scale will the slider come to rest (figure 4). A fit adult can typically achieve a peak flow in excess of 600 litres per minute. Of course this rate is achieved only momentarily – the lungs of an adult can hold between 5 and 6 litres of air in total. Even when we have fully breathed out there is still a bit over a litre of air still in the lungs so it only takes a few seconds for someone who has no chest problems to empty their lungs forcefully of air.

It's important to remember that the peak flow reading is the *fastest* blow, not the longest, so it does require a good effort to get an accurate reading. The technique requires a bit of practice, and the method is as follows:

1. Set the slider to zero and hold the meter so that your fingers are clear of the slot in which the indicator marker runs.
2. Stand up or sit up fully so that your chest movement will be unobstructed.
3. Take a full breath and then close your lips *over* the mouthpiece (don't blow the meter like a trumpet as you won't get your maximum reading that way).
4. Blow hard and fast, then check and write down the reading from the side of the meter.
5. Have a short rest and repeat the reading two more times. Take the best of the three to be your peak flow reading at that time.

Figure 4: Peak flow meter in use

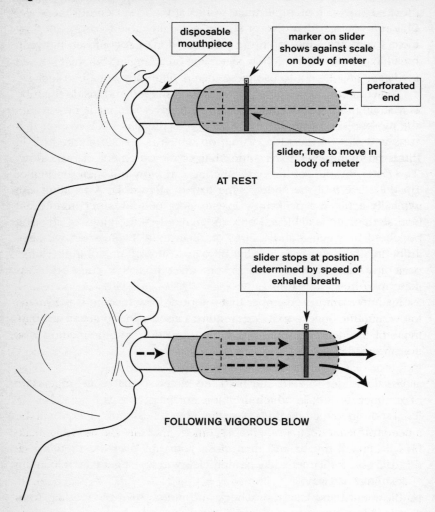

Expected values for peak flow readings vary between individuals, but a few examples are as follows:

- A 25-year-old man 1.85 m (6' 1") tall will have an average PEFR of 635 L/min.
- A 40-year-old woman 1.57 m (5' 2") tall will have an average of 465 L/min.
- A child between six and 15 years old and 1.40 m (4' 7") tall will have an average of 300 L/min.

Patterns of peak flow readings

The solid line in figure 5 shows the pattern of peak flow readings you would expect to see in someone without asthma, who recorded their best peak flow reading twice a day (morning and evening) over a period of a couple of weeks. There is a little fluctuation, probably accounted for by a variation in effort or technique, but generally the peak flow remains quite stable. The dotted line shows a peak flow pattern from someone of comparable build but who has untreated asthma. A typical finding is that the morning peak flow is significantly lower than the evening reading, and that all the readings are lower than those of the non-asthmatic person. This swing between morning and evening readings is called 'diurnal variation' and its presence is a good indicator that asthma control is not at its best, although exactly why asthmatic people show this swing is not fully understood. For the sake of argument a diurnal variation of 20 per cent of peak flow readings or less is considered normal whereas greater variation indicates asthma, or a need for better treatment. The best time to measure the morning peak flow is immediately after rising as this tends to be the lowest reading of the day, and the last reading at night tends to be the highest.

It should become clear during the course of this book that a common predicament these days is deciding whether someone does or does not have asthma, especially if the symptom is just a persistent cough and there are no abnormal signs when the doctor listens to the chest. A 'peak flow diary' kept for a few weeks may reveal diurnal variation of the peak flow and therefore supports the diagnosis of asthma.

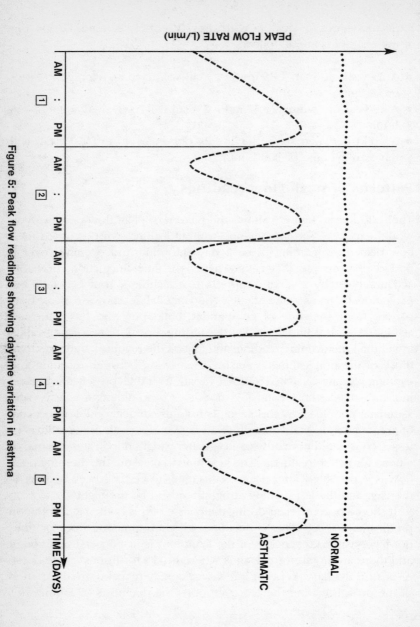

Figure 5: Peak flow readings showing daytime variation in asthma

Further evidence that someone has asthma could be gained by measuring their peak flow before and after a burst of vigorous exercise (provided they are fit enough in general terms to do this). Exercise is a common trigger for asthma and therefore can cause a drop in the peak flow. Deliberately provoking an asthma attack using more specific bronchoconstrictors is not suitable for use in ordinary asthma diagnosis as it requires special expertise and is potentially dangerous. It is however a useful technique in asthma research studies when done under proper supervision.

Even in people with known asthma the peak flow diary can reveal that they are putting up with poorly controlled symptoms. Only after their treatment has subsequently improved do they realise that they've been feeling less well than they should have for some time. A peak flow diary can also be helpful in detecting occupational asthma. If there is a pattern of steady decline in peak flow during the working week and improvement on days off then this suggests exposure at work to something that's triggering an asthma response.

Response to treatment

Asthma is confirmed if there is an improvement in the peak flow following the use of a quick-acting bronchodilator inhaler such as salbutamol. Inhaler treatments are detailed further in chapter 5 but, in brief, quick-acting bronchodilator drugs open up the bronchi within minutes after they are inhaled. A 15 to 20 per cent improvement in the peak flow 20 to 30 minutes after a dose of an appropriate inhaler would be taken as a positive result, i.e. it confirms the 'reversibility' of the bronchial narrowing.

Limitations of PEFR readings

The peak flow reading is easy to measure and requires only simple, inexpensive equipment that almost anyone can learn to use adequately, but it is a test that is prone to error. The reading depends very much on the amount of effort put in to blowing out quickly as well as technique in sealing the lips properly. It is therefore unsuitable for small children, or for someone with poor muscle strength or who finds it difficult to blow out hard for other reasons. Some of these limitations can be overcome by conducting a more sophisticated test of breathing but this requires a more complex piece of equipment called a spirometer that most GPs do not have access to in the surgery.

Diurnal variation does not always show in everyone with asthma – at both ends of the spectrum of severity. Thus, in mild asthma the variation may be too small to be distinguishable from normal, or it may come and go and the test period might coincide with a good spell. In severe asthma the amount of inflammation of the airways can be too much for there to be much variation over the course of a day in the extent of the bronchial narrowing, in which case no diurnal variation is seen, i.e. the peak flow is low all the time. These limitations are relatively minor, and the PEFR reading remains the most useful objective measurement in the routine care of asthma. Every asthmatic person ought to have their own peak flow meter and know how to use it properly.

Chest X-rays

Asthma on its own does not cause abnormal findings to appear on X-ray pictures of the chest, although there are related lung conditions that do show up on a chest X-ray. Generally speaking a chest X-ray is helpful only when looking for information other than to do with asthma. For example, one would usually do a chest X-ray in any adult complaining of a persistent cough for more than a few weeks, even if asthma was the suspected diagnosis, as it is necessary to exclude other possible causes of coughing, including serious conditions such as lung tumours. These other potential diagnoses are very much more common in adults than in children but very occasionally one comes across a child whose cough is due to an inhaled foreign body such as a peanut that has escaped detection until a chest X-ray is done. Also, a chest X-ray would be indicated if there were other significant symptoms that could not be caused by asthma, such as the coughing of blood or the presence of pain on breathing.

A 'routine' chest X-ray is therefore unnecessary in the majority of people with asthma but there are lots of exceptions to the rule and the need for a chest X-ray is very much one that depends on an individual's circumstances. A careful history and clinical examination will usually pick out those people who need one right away, and those who don't respond adequately to treatment in a reasonable period of time will be the majority of the remainder who should have one done.

Blood and 'allergy' tests

There are many dozens of blood tests in common use by doctors but almost none of them are of any value in diagnosing or monitoring asthma. The exceptions are tests related to the immune system and to the detection of allergy in an asthmatic person, and even then there is much potential for confusion. Some of these tests can be done on blood samples but a type of test known as a 'skin prick test' is also potentially very helpful in asthma management. Before we can tackle that topic, a knowledge of the basics of the immune system is required.

Antigens and antibodies

The 'immune system' is a short phrase that covers a highly complex aspect of the function of the body and it is a system of many parts. Everywhere – in the lining of the lungs and digestive system, within organs and tissues, in the blood and in the multiple lymph glands that are connected throughout almost all of the tissues – there are cells capable of detecting proteins that are different from those natural to ourselves. Most often these are bacteria or viruses although sometimes the immune system will attack natural tissues of the body too.

When a foreign protein (called an 'antigen') comes into contact with cells of the immune system these cells produce proteins (called 'antibodies') that fit around the invading antigen in a way that is unique to that particular foreign protein. A fair analogy is of a lock and key, in which the invader is the key and the immune system cells manufacture a lock with which to trap it. The antibody-antigen combination is recognised by other cells within the immune system family that move in and destroy the invader.

The antigen has in this process stimulated the production of a population of immunity cells capable of recognising this antigen again if it invades the body in the future and of manufacturing antibodies against it very quickly the next time round. The length of time this 'memory' effect lasts varies but usually it is many years. This is the principle behind vaccination, in which an inactive protein from, say, measles virus is given as an injection under the skin. This protein is unable to cause a measles infection but it is nonetheless sufficient to make us manufacture antibodies against it, and it acts as a permanent marker for measles virus. Should we at some later date be exposed to measles virus then the antibodies against it circulating in our blood will latch on to it and the antibody-producing cells will also swing into production to produce more of the anti-measles antibody if necessary to overcome the infection.

Asthma and allergy

The relevance of this to asthma is that it isn't just bugs that we can develop antibodies to – there are huge numbers of different proteins in nature that are potentially able to act as allergens. Pollens, moulds, nuts, pet hair and skin, house dust mite droppings, textile fibres, dust and biological washing powders are just a few examples.

What makes these allergens capable of causing symptoms is due to another, slightly more complex way in which this antibody-antigen combination can react in the body of certain people. This is the process that we call allergy, and it is a side shoot of the immune system process that was described above.

IGE AND MAST CELLS
'Immunoglobulin' is the full name for an antibody protein, and is written in shorthand form as 'Ig'. There are several groups of immuno-globulins, identified by an extra letter (IgG, IgM, IgA, IgD and IgE). It is not important to know more about them except that IgE is of particular interest in the problem of allergy. In an allergic person there is usually a large amount of IgE produced by special cells called B cells. This increased IgE can be found in the blood and it can also

attach itself to other cells found in body tissues such as the lungs and skin, called mast cells. When allergens come in contact with the mast cells they attach to the IgE on their surfaces. This reaction triggers a signal into the mast cell causing it to release its chemical contents, such as histamine, into the surrounding tissue. These powerful chemicals cause the tissues to swell and the smooth muscle of the airways to contract, thus narrowing the airway tubes. Other released chemicals attract immune system cells to the inflamed area.

This mechanism involving the mast cells and the release of histamine is now known to be only one of several inflammatory reactions taking place in asthma but it is one of the most important and best understood.

The majority of people, of all ages, who develop asthma are 'atopic', i.e. they have a tendency to develop allergies. Between a third and a half of the general population are atopic to some degree whereas only about one person in five is asthmatic, so there are extra factors involved in determining whether someone becomes asthmatic. More information on these is covered in chapter 3. In very general terms people who develop asthma in childhood tend to be atopic whereas those who develop asthma in later life are not, but there are many exceptions to this. Really what one needs to do is determine whether a particular individual with asthma is or is not also atopic. The easiest way to do this is with skin prick testing.

SKIN PRICK TESTING
The principle behind skin prick testing is very simple. A drop of dilute solution of the substance under test (such as for example an extract of grass pollen) is placed on the skin of the person being tested. The nurse or doctor then pricks the skin under the drop – not enough to cause bleeding but enough so that some of the test solution gets under the skin. Within the skin the substance will provoke an allergic response in people who are sensitive to it, and this shows as a raised lump (weal) surrounded by a larger area of red skin (flare) at the site of the skin prick within about twenty to thirty minutes.

There are several useful points to make about skin prick testing. The technique is easy to carry out and is safe – it is extremely unlikely that a severe allergic reaction will occur in response to a skin prick test, although health professionals who carry out such tests do have to be prepared to deal with a major reaction (called anaphylaxis – see chapter 6). Atopic individuals are fairly easily identified and the tests may show up allergies that were previously not considered important on the basis of the person's experience alone. Skin prick tests can help a lot in deciding on a strategy to reduce the impact of trigger factors in the home, school or work environment.

The tests do also have their limitations. The allergic reaction of interest in asthma is the one taking place within the lung, and a skin test does not measure this directly. Some people react strongly to things that they really are not allergic to (false positive result) and others do not react against things that they know they are allergic to (false negative result). Skin prick tests are unreliable in young children (below four), whose immune systems are still immature (nor do they much appreciate being pricked by needles!). These are minor limitations, however, and the value of skin prick tests much outweighs their disadvantages.

Despite this fact it is very likely that if you are a UK reader with asthma you will probably never have had skin prick testing, or even have discussed it with your doctor or nurse. The reason is the very poor availability of allergy testing within the NHS. Allergy testing kits are fairly expensive, and this is a cost that cannot be recovered by your GP from the NHS. Most of all, skin prick tests take time and in the ever more pressured environment of the NHS, things that take up time are more likely to be short-circuited or left out. Some GPs are interested in allergy testing and can offer it to their patients, and some hospital asthma clinics do allergy testing on the people referred to them. Most people who might benefit from the knowledge gained from allergy tests just get left out. Part of the reason may also be that 'allergy testing' as a concept has been hijacked by some of the least credible forms of alternative medicine, whose methods have little or nothing to do with the immune system. Some health professionals have consequently confused proper allergy testing with quackery and ended up recommending neither.

By the time you have read through the rest of this book you should have a fair idea if allergy testing would be useful to you – generally the answer is yes, especially if you are willing and able to act upon the results (chapter 4). In any case it is worth checking with your GP if it is available locally. If not then a reasonable alternative is a form of blood testing that essentially looks for the presence of IgE antibodies to the major asthma triggers such as pollens and animal proteins. The technical name for these is 'RAST' tests and they should be available to most or all GPs through their local hospital laboratory service. Blood tests are quick to perform at the GP end of the process but more involved and expensive at the laboratory end. They are less sensitive than skin tests and because of their expense usually only a small range of allergens are tested for within the NHS. It is also possible to have allergy tests done by reputable 'allergists', who usually have to be seen privately: contact details are in appendix C.

Common allergens revealed by skin prick or blood tests include:

- Insects – house dust mite is by far the commonest in the UK and Europe but cockroaches are seen in many poorer social settings, and are especially common in the USA.
- Animals – cats are the main culprits but dogs, mice, horses and other animals are also involved. The allergens are present in the animals' coats and saliva.
- Plants – fungi are present both outdoors and indoors in everyone's homes. *Aspergillus* is the name of the commonest one indoors. Pollen from trees (early spring), grasses (late spring and summer) and weeds (summer and autumn) are common allergens.

It is unusual for someone with asthma to be allergic to just one thing – usually there are many factors, although at any time of the year a different one may be the most important. It can therefore be surprisingly difficult for an asthmatic person to be sure what it is that sparks off their asthma most – often as the year rolls by one trigger factor is imperceptibly replaced by another so it is hard to pick out peaks and troughs and thereby trace back to particular triggers.

More information on allergens and how to deal with them is in chapter 4.

Difficulties in diagnosis

Asthma can be easy to diagnose, or very difficult, or somewhere in between. In a few particular groups of asthmatic people the problems are well recognised:

CHILDREN

It was stated earlier that cough and wheeze are common problems in early childhood, and the younger the child the less likely it is that asthma is the cause of these symptoms. For example, babies are prone to bring back feeds, and wheeze and cough can be caused by milk spilling over into the airways instead of being completely swallowed. Other children whose wheeze is caused by a virus infection of the airways (itself a very common occurrence) will wheeze but do not go on to be asthmatic when older. Asthma can be a label that is hard to remove, so it should be applied with care. This also implies that one should look for alternative explanations for the symptoms, but perhaps most importantly it needs to be remembered that even if a child is not 'definitely asthmatic' they can benefit from the treatment for asthma. It is still a common mistake for children to be repeatedly treated with useless antibiotics for wheezy episodes brought on by virus infections. Antibiotics do not kill viruses and they certainly do not relieve bronchospasm. Therefore, instead of being over-careful with the diagnosis of asthma to the extent that the child is inappropriately or ineffectively treated it is better to treat 'as if' asthma is present. Usually this will help the child improve more quickly, and time will tell if asthma is really the underlying problem. Children as young as four can be taught to use a peak flow meter quite well, and junior versions of these meters are available for this purpose.

ELDERLY

Many things conspire to obscure asthma in the elderly. Other conditions such as heart problems can cause breathlessness and wheeze, longstanding smoking may cause lung damage that masks the presence of asthma alongside it and perhaps as much as anything there is a tendency for old age itself to be accepted as a cause of ill health. Even if asthma is suspected it may be necessary for other co-existing problems such as heart failure to be corrected first before the asthma can be revealed or treated. Increasingly there is a tendency to look for asthma in older people and also to try the effect of asthma treatment in people with the main other adult lung condition – chronic obstructive pulmonary (airways) disease (COPD). Until fairly recently COPD has been taken to be a non-reversible lung disease in which airways become blocked due to damage from (usually) cigarette smoking. Although many people who have COPD do not get much help from asthma-type treatment, some do and therefore it is important to consider a trial of this treatment, especially as the distinction between COPD and asthma is not always a clear one. COPD is covered in more detail in chapter 8.

OCCUPATIONAL ASTHMA

According to the Health and Safety Executive (HSE) up to 3,000 people each year in the UK develop asthma as a result of exposure at work to materials that can cause the condition, and this risk can be almost entirely eliminated by proper precautions to protect workers. There are some occupations in which asthma is well known to be a possible 'risk of the job'. For example, paints called isocyanates used particularly in the spray painting of cars have a high tendency to cause asthma if used in poorly ventilated areas and without protective breathing gear. Over 350 agents are officially recognised as potentially able to cause occupational asthma and we can safely assume that this list is incomplete. The degree of hazard can be reduced by good ventilation, avoiding poor working practices and by using effective breathing masks, but in many badly regulated work environments such protection is often unavailable, or just not used. Companies large enough to have their own occupational health service will usually be well aware of the potential risks and will offer adequate protection to their employees. Workers not so lucky may need to seek help from their doctor, trade union or the HSE if occupational asthma is suspected. Proving a cause and effect relationship in the eyes of the law when someone develops asthma at work can be a long, difficult and expensive business that is prone to failure. On the other hand a successful claim will prove expensive to a culpable employer. Occupational asthma should be suspected if asthma symptoms are episodic and show improvement during holidays and particularly if someone works in a known high-risk occupation. Some examples of these are in table 1 and a complete list is available on-line at http://www.asmanet.com/asmapro/jobs.htm#start.

Table 1: Some occupations associagted with asthma

Occupation/industry	Agents causing asthma
Bakers	Flour, enzymes
Electronics	Solder fumes (pine resin or colophony)
Farmers	Organic dusts, mites
Food processing	Shellfish, egg proteins, enzymes, coffee bean dust, tea
Hairdressers	Hairspray
Hospital workers, nurses	Disinfectants, latex
Joiners and sawmill workers	Wood dust, resins
Paint spraying	Ethanolamine, isocyanates
Plastics industry	Organic chemicals
Poultry workers	Poultry mites, droppings, feathers
Rubber processing	Formaldehyde, ethylene diamine
Welders	Stainless steel fumes, chromium salts

COUGH-VARIANT ASTHMA

This is the term for people whose symptom is only that of a cough. The cough is due to asthma, but people with it do not wheeze and they can be very difficult to diagnose. Often someone with cough-variant asthma will develop the cough first after an upper airways infection. Perhaps after a week or two of getting tired out coughing all the time they will go along to their GP, who on the basis of thinking this may be a bronchitis infection prescribes an antibiotic – but it fails to work. Weeks or months can pass with the cough going on and on, particularly at night. Meantime the careful GP will have arranged a chest X-ray to exclude other problems in the lung – and it comes back normal. Only by considering the possibility of cough-variant asthma will the correct treatment be prescribed and the cough relieved. Fortunately most doctors are now wise to this type of asthma and are quicker to spot it and treat it properly. Peak flow tests can be helpful in diagnosing it by showing the variation in peak flow, especially at night, but often the only way to diagnose it is to prescribe an effective course of asthma treatment and to then see what happens to the patient's symptoms.

Severity of asthma

It isn't enough just to say that asthma is or is not present. By classifying the severity of the asthma one can pitch the treatment at the right level. Under-treatment causes the asthmatic person to experience more symptoms than they should have, as well as exposing them to the risk of getting a severe asthma attack. Over-treatment leads to more side effects than are necessary from the medicines. The severity grades for asthma are dealt with more fully in the chapter on treatment plans (chapter 6).

SUMMARY
- The typical symptoms of asthma are cough, wheeze and breathlessness.
- Not all of these symptoms need to be present in an asthmatic person at any one time.
- Asthma is diagnosed mostly on the basis of a person's history of symptoms plus the findings on medical examination.
- The peak expiratory flow rate (PEFR) is a simple measure of the degree of narrowing of the airways and can be used in diagnosing asthma. It is particularly useful in monitoring asthma.

- In untreated asthma the morning PEFR reading is typically lower than the evening reading.
- Most people with asthma are atopic, i.e. they have a tendency to develop allergic reactions to certain substances.
- Skin prick tests are the easiest way to detect atopic individuals, and to reveal which are the main factors possibly triggering their asthma.
- Asthma is commonest in children, in whom it can also be difficult to diagnose, especially in the very young.
- Asthma is under-recognised in the elderly.
- Occupational asthma should be considered in someone who develops asthma in adulthood, especially if they do not have a background tendency to allergies.
- Cough-variant asthma is that in which cough is the main or only symptom. It can easily be mistaken as 'bronchitis' initially but responds only to asthma treatment.

Chapter 3

The Causes of Asthma

It was mentioned in the last chapter that asthma tends to occur in 'atopic' people – but not all of them, and it also occurs in people with no previous history of allergic reactions. We've seen that there are many recognised substances that are associated with occupational asthma, but that still doesn't answer the question of what causes asthma in the first place. We also need to explain why asthma is becoming increasingly common in our society.

Cells of the immune system

Asthma is now one of the most intensely researched areas of medicine and a vast body of knowledge has been accumulated about it. In common with every other area of medical knowledge the complete picture is for future generations to fully comprehend, but we are a long way down the road to achieving that understanding now. It's clear from examining lung tissue in asthma that many inflammatory cells gather within the bronchi and stay there, and that this is the primary cause of the condition.

There are several groups of cells dispersed throughout the body that are members of the immune system and of particular interest in asthma are those known as lymphocytes. Lymphocytes, like most such cells, originate mainly in the bone marrow and then undergo further change to divide into two sub-groups – the 'T' and the 'B' lymphocytes. Most lymphocytes in the blood are 'T' cells and they are capable of a multitude of different actions such as the destruction of other cells or the development of other immune reactions. B lymphocytes are specially designed to manufacture antibody proteins. T and B cells are present in the bloodstream, in most tissues and in particular within the lymph nodes. Lymph nodes are distributed widely within the abdomen and the chest but also can sometimes be felt in more superficial areas such as under the armpits or at the sides of the neck during an infection. Within the lymph nodes the T and B cells continuously undergo multiplication and sorting into their individual roles. Between them, the T and B lymphocytes form the backbone of the immune family of cells.

When an antigen gets into the body in the way already described, T cells become activated to produce signalling chemicals (called cytokines) that send messages to other immune system cells and B cells are triggered to produce IgE.

The combination of released cytokines and IgE stimulates mast cells to release histamine and causes other inflammatory cells (particularly those called eosinophils) to get involved locally too. The result is the swelling of bronchi, shedding of surface lining cells, increased mucus production, thickening of smooth muscle in the walls of the bronchi and all the other features that make up the observed changes in asthma.

A great deal more information than this is known about the roles of other immune system cells and the various biochemical processes that go on between them in allergic conditions. Such knowledge has led to newer treatments for asthma and much more is hoped to come from such research. It is a complex area to understand and fortunately we can skip past most of it in our overview.

Risk factors for asthma

Knowledge of the factors that are associated with the later development of asthma is a major area of interest for two reasons. One is that such knowledge should throw further light on the reasons why asthma develops, but secondly, and in a more practical sense, provided the risk factors can be changed, this gives us a method of making asthma less common or at least of reducing its impact.

Risk factors can be divided into two main groups:

1. Those factors that are particular to the individual (called 'host factors'). These are:
   - genetic inheritance, including male or female sex
   - tendency to atopy (allergy) and bronchial 'hyper-responsiveness'.
2. Environmental factors. These influence the development of asthma in people with a tendency to get it:
   - indoor allergens (insect and animal allergens, fungi)
   - outdoor allergens (pollens, fungi)
   - occupational agents
   - tobacco smoke (both active and passive smoking)
   - air pollution
   - airway infections
   - drug therapy
   - socio-economic status
   - family size (asthma is commoner in small families).

Host factors

GENETICS

The children of someone with asthma are more likely to become asthmatic than the children of a non-asthmatic. Such a relationship could of course be partially explained by the fact that child and parent usually live in the same household and are therefore exposed to the same trigger factors for asthma, but there is other evidence to show that the link is really through the genes and not just the shared conditions at home. For example, twins who are raised apart show a much higher likelihood of both being asthmatic, despite living in different home situations. Genes are the individual units of hereditary information that are stored in great numbers in our chromosomes – the rod-shaped pairs of genetic material present within the nucleus of almost all of our cells. Many types of gene differences are now recognised in connection with specific diseases, but no single gene 'fault' has been found to be associated with asthma. Instead it seems certain that there are many possible combinations of gene patterns, which, in the right circumstances, can predispose a person to becoming asthmatic. For those who like to know the details, there are 23 pairs of chromosomes in each of our cells. Genes that seem to be involved in asthma and allergy have been found on chromosome numbers 6, 11, 12, 13, 14 and 19. Undoubtedly the amount of new information that will be discovered in this area over the next few years will be substantial.

GENDER

In childhood, asthma is more common in boys than in girls. By the age of ten the sexes are about equal and then at puberty females overtake males and stay that way into adulthood. Some of these differences are thought to be related to differences in the sizes of the airways – boys having smaller airways in childhood than girls but larger airways when mature.

RACE

It is possible that racial origin pays some part in determining a person's tendency to develop asthma but there is more evidence to suggest that it is the socio-economic status of different racial or ethnic groups that is the real cause of the differences observed. More economically disadvantaged groups have higher numbers of asthmatic people. Other factors that could be important are different diets and exposure patterns to allergens.

ATOPIC TENDENCY

This is really a specific aspect of gene inheritance. Some of the genes involved in the manufacture within cells of proteins involved in inflammation have been identified and show inheritance patterns that link them to the risk of becoming asthmatic.

Environmental factors

ALLERGENS

There is a good deal of unresolved debate in current medical circles about the importance of how much exposure to allergens in infancy affects an individual's chances of later becoming allergic and/or asthmatic. It could be the case, if someone is exposed in the first few months of life to lots of allergens, that this primes the immune system to develop allergies when older. In fact, research on the blood of babies newly born to atopic mothers shows that their lymphocytes are already capable of reacting against common allergens such as house dust mite. This suggests, therefore, that the process of becoming sensitive to allergens actually starts in the womb and many experts are of the opinion that asthma is a condition that always has its roots in very early childhood or pre-birth. As yet the evidence for such theories is weak. It is likely to be correct, though, that high exposure to allergens in the first year or two of life will increase the likelihood of developing allergies later, and sometimes this will show itself as asthma.

The facts that modern houses tend to be carpeted, well insulated from draughts (and therefore get less fresh air than old, leaky houses) and centrally heated, which in turn encourages the growth of the house dust mite (see later in this chapter), are often quoted as possible reasons why we now see increasing rates of asthma. Poorer households also tend to be more prone to harbour mites in older carpets and upholstered furniture. In atopic people of any age these factors increase the likelihood of getting asthma.

AIRWAY INFECTIONS

In any age group infection of the bronchi can cause temporary wheezing. This is seen often by general practitioners and it can be difficult to distinguish a wheeze and cough lasting some weeks following an airways infection from the 'cough-variant asthma' described in the previous chapter. There may not actually be very much difference. Recurrent viral infection of the airways is commonplace in childhood and 30 per cent of infants get wheezy in their first year. The risk of later development of asthma is greatest in infants who get an airway infection with a virus called Respiratory Syncytial Virus (RSV). RSV doesn't always infect the lower airways (bronchi) – sometimes it just causes a cold – but when it does go into the bronchi in this age group it causes an illness called bronchiolitis. Most infants with bronchiolitis need a brief hospital admission but recover perfectly well, but they are more likely to be asthmatic by school age. They are also more likely to have a family history of allergy.

TOBACCO SMOKE

There is no doubt that exposure of children to tobacco smoke markedly increases their chances of getting upper airways infections, blocked ears due to excess catarrh ('glue ear') and asthma. As with other allergens, the process may start in the womb if the mother smokes. Smoking in the mother is more strongly related than smoking in the father to the development of asthma in a child, possibly because of the link in pregnancy and also perhaps because the father is more likely to be out working when the child is young and therefore his smoking has less impact on the child than that of the mother, who is in greater contact with the child. Anyone smoking at home where there is a child will have an adverse effect upon that child's health, as well as their own.

Tobacco smoke contains over 4,000 substances, many of which are highly irritant and damaging to the sensitive lining of the airways. Passive smoking in both children and adults is proved to be just as harmful as active smoking and the ability to breathe clean air should really be seen as a fundamental human right.

The impact of smoking on the adult asthmatic has been well studied and is not good news for the person concerned. Such adults have a markedly increased rate of lung damage compared to asthmatics who do not smoke; they also get more severe asthma attacks and have poorer response to asthma treatments. Stopping smoking is therefore an overriding priority for anyone with asthma. There is much help available for someone who wishes to stop smoking. Some relevant contacts in this regard are listed in appendix C. A companion book in this series also details methods on how to stop.

OCCUPATIONAL EXPOSURE AND AIR POLLUTION

The types of job associated with asthma were covered in chapter 2, along with some of the known agents that can cause it. There are plenty of substances yet to be added to that list for which the evidence is yet to be gathered.

Air pollution has multiple components – both outdoors and indoors. Outdoors the main irritants are sulphur dioxide and ozone released by industrial plants, and the gases and very fine particles released by car engines. Exhaust from poorly designed or maintained car (diesel) engines contains particles that can attract other allergens such as pollen, thus increasing their delivery to the bronchi. While not necessarily causing asthma directly, such pollution worsens pre-existing asthma.

Indoor pollution is important because of the amount of time people spend inside buildings. Cooking and heating appliances using gas, wood, coal or oil produce various irritant gases. Air is re-circulated more often when windows are kept shut and many of the materials and glues used in modern building materials and furniture construction can release fumes that worsen asthma.

DRUG THERAPY

Some drugs can directly or indirectly act upon the bronchial tubes to narrow them and thereby cause or worsen asthma. Beta-blockers are widely used medicines for the treatment of high blood pressure and angina but a common side effect in susceptible individuals is that they cause the muscles of the bronchial tubes to contract, so narrowing the airways. This is a direct effect of the drug and not an allergic reaction. Beta-blockers should be avoided in people with known asthma but sometimes a person with hitherto unrecognised asthma gets wheezy when started on a beta-blocker in good faith. Usually the wheeze goes away when the beta-blocker is stopped. It is not a good idea to keep taking a beta-blocker and use asthma treatment to deal with the wheeze – an alternative to the beta-blocker should be found. Beta-blockers should however not be stopped abruptly without a doctor's advice.

A small but significant number of people are allergic to aspirin and develop a wheeze when they take it. People with 'aspirin-sensitive asthma' are often also allergic to anti-inflammatory painkillers of the ibuprofen family (e.g. fenbufen, flurbiprofen, diclofenac). Collectively these drugs are called non-steroidal anti-inflammatory drugs, or NSAIDs. Aspirin and NSAIDs are therefore best avoided by people with asthma but this is not always convenient. NSAIDs are, for example, commonly needed to relieve the discomfort of arthritis – which is more common than asthma especially in older people. So sometimes it is acceptable for an asthmatic person to try a NSAID. If there is no obvious reaction then it can be continued but one should remain alert to the fact that sensitivity to the NSAID might develop at a later date and be ready to stop the drug if the asthma begins to worsen. Ibuprofen is currently the only NSAID that can be bought in the UK from a pharmacist (or supermarket) without a doctor's prescription. It is always a good policy for someone with asthma to check with a pharmacist or with their doctor if they intend to take an over-the-counter remedy of any type as some others are also best avoided.

Aspirin's correct name is acetylsalicylic acid, and related compounds called salicylates are widely present in foodstuffs. It is sometimes worthwhile for someone who is known to be aspirin-sensitive to exclude salicylates from his or her diet for a while to see if it helps improve their asthma. It may not, and a salicylate-free diet is not easy to maintain long-term so it is not an experiment worth persevering with unless it gives obvious results. A dietician is the best person to advise on such diets, and you can be referred to one by your GP.

STRESS

Stress is a factor often cited as a cause of other conditions, such as skin problems, irritable bowel syndrome, hair loss, cystitis and many others, including asthma. It is very difficult to measure someone's degree of stress in a meaningful way and studies on stress in relation to other conditions therefore have to be treated with some caution. Stress can come from many different directions, including unsatisfactory relationships, financial and work-related problems, depression, alcoholism and other types of ill health. In turn these might cause someone to neglect their asthma treatment or avoid seeking help for it if it begins to worsen. Stress is unlikely to cause asthma but it can be a contributing factor in poorly controlled asthma.

FAMILY SIZE

Children with no or only one sibling are more likely to get asthma than those with two or more older siblings. Somehow the exposure of young children to older children in the same family reduces their likelihood of becoming wheezy.

THE 'HYGIENE HYPOTHESIS'

One of the most obvious aspects of living in Western society is that hygiene and sanitation levels are generally higher than in developing countries. Foods are often sterile or very nearly so, and packaged to keep them that way. 'Germs' are seen as the enemy and if one were to believe the advertising industry civilisation would pretty much come to an abrupt end if it were not for the sterling efforts of the disinfectant manufacturers. That this is patently rubbish is clear from a moment's reflection on the length of time mankind has survived cheek by jowl with all manner of microbes. It is of course also true that food and water-borne disease is still the scourge of much of the world's population who do not have access to clean water and waste disposal systems, but our modern Western obsession with cleanliness is a possible explanation for the upsurge in allergic conditions. Much of our experience of the world, in an immune sense, comes from what we take in to our bodies in the form of food. The immune system of the gut is highly sophisticated, and the theory is that normally we would de-sensitise ourselves to allergens by the constant re-exposure we'd get through eating a less sanitised diet. In the event, by ingesting so many fewer microbes than we used to we develop a reverse tendency to react with more allergic illnesses to those allergens that we do meet. Put another way, infections seem to stimulate a type of immunity that protects against the development of allergies and asthma.

There are several pieces of supportive evidence for this 'hygiene hypothesis'. For example, people who grow up on a farm and are therefore in regular contact with animals are less likely to become atopic than the average city dweller. In a study of Italian military students those who had antibodies to Hepatitis A, a viral infection of the liver usually obtained from contaminated food, were less likely to be atopic than those who had no antibodies to the virus. If someone has antibodies then they must have had previous exposure to the virus (although they would not necessarily have had the full hepatitis illness). The presence of Hepatitis A antibodies was therefore taken to be a marker of childhood contact with infections in general. Of further interest in this study was the finding that having antibodies to Hepatitis A virus was unimportant in deciding if someone became atopic if they also had three or more older siblings. If the hygiene hypothesis is correct, this would be because of the extra bugs brought in to the household by several older children.

Attendance at pre-school nursery is an excellent way to pick up infections from other children. According to the hygiene hypothesis this would be expected to reduce a child's likelihood of becoming atopic; however this has not been consistently shown to be true. The infection theory is therefore not watertight. No one is advocating that eating dirt is a way to treat asthma, and it should also be clear by now that a bacteria-free childhood is only one of the possibly relevant links between allergy and affluence, but it may be one of the most important ones.

HOUSE DUST MITE

The humble house dust mite is the commonest indoor allergen capable of causing asthma. Not every asthmatic person is allergic to it, and measures to control house dust mite can easily go 'over the top' without necessarily improving asthma (see next chapter), but it does deserve a special mention.

House dust mites are tiny – about 0.3 mm long, so you need very good eyesight to see them without a magnifying glass. They are arachnids, so are in the same biological class as spiders and scorpions. They are present everywhere – having mites in your house does not imply that your house is dirty. House dust mites settle on clothes, furniture, bedding, carpets, curtains – in fact anywhere that dust can settle. The commonest type of house dust mite in the UK has the grand sounding and nearly unpronounceable full title of *Dermatophagoides pteronyssinus*. Human skin scales are its favoured food – and they can get by on very little. It's completely normal for human beings to shed dead skin cells from the top layer of the skin – each of us loses about 1 gram of skin daily this way. This is enough to feed 10,000 house dust mites for six months! *Dermatophagoides farinae* is the other main species of mite in the UK and it feeds on flour and biscuit crumbs.

Mites do not drink – they absorb moisture from the air, so they prefer warm, humid environments. They also cannot eat dry skin scales – the scales first have to be partially broken down by microbes such as fungi and yeasts. These too will thrive best in moist, warm, poorly ventilated places. A damp British house with the windows shut and the heating on full blast does very nicely, thank you, and carpets, beds and soft furnishings are the ideal hiding places.

The individual house dust mite lives for about three months and its faeces are actually what contain the allergens (which are proteins called Der P1 and Der P2). Mite droppings therefore persist and cause allergic reactions long after the mite has died. Measures to reduce house dust mite irritation, as we'll see shortly, therefore need both to kill the organism and to remove the allergens. An additional mechanism by which house dust mite causes asthma is that it produces enzymes which can break through the lining cells of the bronchi. This exposes the underlying layers, increasing the penetration of antigen into the tissues and contributing to the shedding of lining cells that is seen in asthma.

SUMMARY

- The causes of asthma are not fully understood but key processes include the involvement of T and B lymphocyte cells triggered by inhalation of antigen.
- Other agents that provoke asthma do so by means other than through immune reactions. These act directly on the bronchi to inflame the linings and trigger bronchospasm. Tobacco and many of the substances responsible for occupational asthma act this way.
- A minority of people with asthma are allergic to aspirin and NSAID painkillers. These drugs should therefore be used with care in asthma.
- Beta-blockers are commonly used drugs for high blood pressure and angina, and they can cause or worsen asthma in susceptible people.
- Asthma has a genetic component but there is no single gene pattern associated with it. Instead many different gene combinations can give rise to asthma if other factors, such as exposure to certain antigens, also occur.
- The timing of antigen exposure may be important to the development of asthma. The vulnerable period is likely to be in infancy or even prior to birth, through exposure in the mother.
- Childhood airway infection, especially by Respiratory Syncytial Virus, increases the chance of later becoming asthmatic.
- It is possible that reduced childhood exposure to microbes accounts for at least some of the increase in allergic diseases such as asthma seen over the past 30 years.
- House dust mite is the commonest indoor allergen in the UK and thrives best in warm humid conditions.

Chapter 4

Treating Asthma (1) – Minimising Trigger Factors

Asthma has to be considered a condition for which drug therapy is usually required, but it makes sense to minimise the need for treatment in everyone. That means doing as much as possible to identify and eliminate irritants and environmental causes. In this chapter we'll consider what can reasonably be done in the domestic situation without going overboard. Occupational asthma is a topic beyond the scope of this book and dealing with it is left to the specialist in occupational medicine, although from time to time it'll be mentioned again.

There is a great deal of information available on gadgets to remove dust from the air, special mattresses, bedding, pillows, furniture and all manner of other items meant to be helpful in asthma, and not all of this information is accurate. Much of it comes from the manufacturers of the items concerned, who might not be considered the most impartial sources of information. Many of these items are expensive, so before spending lots of money and effort on possibly ineffective solutions it makes sense to look at what can reasonably be done and for those actions which have some evidence of efficacy.

Identify trigger factors

For this you can start with a pen and paper. If you have had asthma for any length of time it is likely that you will already know some or many items or situations that make your asthma worse. This will not always mean that you can avoid them (for example it would be poor asthma treatment if you had to stop exercising) but it will be an excellent starting point for identifying which factors you can tackle most easily.

Write down a list of possible irritants relevant to yourself, and make a note the next time you get an asthma attack of anything you might have been in contact with that could have been responsible. Generally this means anything you could have inhaled, but food sensitivity can also trigger asthma, so it is worth noting what you have eaten too. As we'll see later the cause and effect relationship between food reactions and asthma attacks is less well established and also is delayed, so it can be quite difficult to identify culpable foods. Asthma reactions to inhaled irritants generally come on more quickly after exposure and are easier to spot (as always there are plenty of exceptions to this rule, and it is possible for an asthma trigger to be something that you've been exposed to for years without realising it has been causing symptoms).

To help you, here is a starting list of possible triggers:

- tobacco smoke
- perfume and aftershave lotions
- air freshener, hairspray or other aerosols
- changes in air temperature
- exposure to animals, birds, flowers, cut grass
- domestic chores like bed changing or vacuuming
- hobby interests (woodworking, electronic circuit construction, model making, gardening)

- DIY activities
- exercise
- stressful or exciting situations
- colds and other airway infections
- traffic pollution
- work place triggers.

Identify atopy

This topic has already been touched upon several times. Atopy means a tendency to develop allergic reactions and many of the symptoms people get after inhaling trigger substances are allergy-based rather than due to direct irritation from toxic substances. Skin prick tests can reveal substances not previously noticed to be trigger factors, and history taking is unlikely to be reliable enough in children to identify all important trigger factors. However, this doesn't mean that everyone with asthma needs skin prick tests – one can apply a few guidelines to narrow this down.

The more of the questions below to which the answer is 'yes', the more likely it is that you have atopic asthma and therefore skin prick testing (or RAST blood testing) will be useful to you:

- Your asthma started in childhood.
- Your symptoms are worse in bed, in old or damp houses, in the winter (when the heating is on), after vacuuming or dusting, when sitting in old furniture or in houses with fitted carpets. All of these indicate house dust mite sensitivity.
- Your symptoms are worse depending on the season – spring, summer or autumn, or after cutting long grass, after exposure to plants or otherwise related to pollen (check in the newspapers when pollen counts are high and see if this ties up with your bad spells).
- You get symptoms if raking up leaves or cut grass that's been left for a while, in damp or musty houses or in winter, all of which make it likely that you are reacting to mould.
- You have a cat or dog and notice symptoms related to animal exposure or when cleaning out guinea pig or rabbit hutches, bird cages, etc.
- You are sensitive to aspirin or NSAID drugs like ibuprofen.

If none of the above applies to you then it is pretty unlikely you are an atopic individual. Your asthma is more likely to be due to the direct effects of noxious irritants such as those encountered in occupational asthma or from tobacco smoke.

If you do seem to be atopic on the basis of your experience then skin prick testing should be your next step if you can arrange it. A concerted attack on eliminating house dust mite will after all take up a fair bit of your time, energy and at least some of your money, and if you are not allergic to dust mite then that will not be the best use of your resources! Allowing for the fact that skin prick tests are not infallible they can nevertheless point you in the right direction. You may get a full house of positive reactions against virtually every test substance, in which case you will at least know that what you are going for is the minimisation of allergen exposure and not its complete removal (an impossible goal). On the other hand you might strike it lucky and identify one or two strongly positive triggers that you can take steps to eliminate effectively. If that happens to be the family moggie, then you may have some serious thinking to do.

Stop smoking

For any asthmatic person who smokes the single most effective way that they can help themselves is to stop smoking. Nothing else really comes close. Not only does smoking accelerate the rate of lung damage that can occur in long-standing asthma but it also increases the risk of heart disease, hardening of the arteries and lung cancer. Passive smoking is just as bad and if you have to tolerate this at work you really should be complaining about it very vigorously.

If your partner smokes then try hard to persuade him or her to give up with you, as your chances of mutual success will be magnified. Seek help in the form of more information and see if there are stop smoking clinics in your area. There should be, and your GP ought to be able to refer you to one. Nicotine replacement therapy is available with and without a prescription and bupropion (Zyban) is an alternative drug that can help break the nicotine addiction that keeps you smoking.

It is essential to keep cigarette smoke away from children, but especially so for children with asthma. Exposing children to cigarette smoke is completely unjustified and in fact neglectful. Having a puff in the room next door is useless – cigarette smoke permeates easily through a house. If you really can't give up then smoke outside, but keep trying, as on average it takes someone five tries to finally pack in the habit.

House dust mite

If, as is likely, you are allergic to house dust mite then you have to tackle it. You can go to extremes and strip your house of carpets, replacing them with wood floors or vinyl, replace all your upholstered furniture with leather, replace your bedding with new stuff covered in mite-free covers, replace all other soft furnishings and spend a lot of time cleaning out every cupboard, nook and cranny in the house. Of course, it would be best to get someone else (who isn't asthmatic) to do all of this while you stay elsewhere until it's all over. It's quite likely that such a comprehensive clean-up will dramatically reduce the amount of house dust mite material in the house and will probably improve your symptoms, although it is a bit of a gamble as few people have only a single allergy. Perhaps there are some people who can afford to do all of this, but it is neither essential nor practical to go this far for the majority. The following list of things to do should however be seen as the minimum that will make a difference:

BEDDING
At night we spend on average eight hours in contact with house dust mite allergen. Beds are warm, pillows can become damp from our breath, and mattresses damp from sweat or from bed-wetting in childhood are ideal mite territory. Mite-proof covers for the pillows, mattress and duvet can be re-used time and again after washing (at 60 degrees C – mites are killed above 55 degrees C). Replacing a pillow is cheap, and using mite-proof covers from new will reduce the build-up of mites within the pillow subsequently. National pharmacy

chains now sell these covers, but they can also be obtained on-line. Information on these products is kept up to date by the British Allergy Foundation (see appendix C). Synthetic pillows are not necessarily better than feather ones unless you have an allergy to feathers. Mites don't mind living with modern fibres.

Do not air or vacuum the mattress as this just stirs up clouds of allergen. The mites are inside the mattress and won't be blown away in the wind or sucked up the vacuum cleaner pipe. It is, however, essential to dry a mattress thoroughly if it gets wet. Protective covers should be used if a child is bed-wetting. One can spend an awful lot of money on fancy mattresses that the manufacturers claim will do wonders for your back. The human spine is a pretty strong item and not easily damaged by an economy-priced mattress that you can afford to replace more often than an expensive one.

SOFT FURNISHINGS AND TOYS

Replace curtains in bedrooms with blinds or machine-washable (hot cycle) material. Do this before replacing the bed linen or allergens released from the curtains will fall on to the new mite-proof bed covers! Throw out unwanted soft toys, cloth books and the like. Soft toys that have to stay should be frozen to kill off the mites and then washed to remove the allergens. Drying them off thoroughly is essential – the best way to do that is in the tumble dryer. Freezing should be repeated every week or two.

Mite-proof covers can sometimes be obtained for furniture although they are of dubious benefit. Particularly in the case of old upholstered furniture one really needs to look seriously at letting it go and replacing it instead with vinyl or leather-covered furniture. Most people's finances prevent this being a priority.

CARPETS

Mites thrive in the depths of carpets. Some modern vacuum cleaners are very efficient at removing dust particles and mite-sized material but very few cleaners have been subjected to study in the medical sense. The Medivac cleaner is one that has and is effective in removing dust while not at the same time kicking up allergens into the air – a fault most conventional cleaners are guilty of. Many of the most recent vacuum cleaners are sold as allergy-friendly on the basis that their filtering systems are effective at removing small particles. This is likely to be correct but the lack of scientific information in this area makes it impossible to provide any meaningful list of 'best buys'. Check at least that the cleaner has a built-in filter capable of catching very fine particles (these are called HEPA filters – high efficiency particulate air filters). The 'cyclone' type of bag-free cleaner is potentially able to pick up extremely small dust particles, but they are not all equally effective. The most technically efficient are those manufactured by Dyson® but as yet there is no published information that proves these are better for asthmatic people. Emptying cleaners is a job that should be delegated when possible to someone who is lucky enough not to be asthmatic.

Unfortunately good cleaners tend to be expensive, and since it is necessary to repeatedly clean a carpet it is not economic or effective to hire such machines for occasional use. One possibility, though, is for a few families with asthmatic members to get together and purchase a cleaner that they can share between them.

The most effective way to clean a carpet of mite material is to steam clean it. This destroys the protein in the mite faeces that causes the allergy in the first place. Such steam cleaners are again not cheap but as they need to be used only once every few months the possibility of hiring one or sharing one between several households is more practical.

VENTILATION AND HUMIDITY
In an often cold and damp climate such as in Britain it is understandable that people prefer to keep their windows closed and the heating on. Such conditions also raise the humidity of the air, which favours the growth of mould and house dust mites. Getting used to more fresh air and cooler homes can benefit asthma. Mites cannot survive in extremely dry air, so a powerful de-humidifier can reduce mite populations if used over a long enough period of time, but these are expensive to buy.

Animals

Logic tends to go out the window when it comes to the family pet. All furry warm-blooded animals are potentially prone to generate allergens in the form of dander and in their saliva and urine but many families retain their pet even when it is known that it is responsible for allergic reactions (about a third of asthmatic people are allergic to cats alone). Getting rid of the pet may not make an immediate difference as the allergens produced by cats for example can linger for many months after the cat has been removed. There is little in the way of helpful advice one can give someone with asthma who prefers to retain a pet he is allergic to, but the following points may be useful:

- Air filters (HEPA filters) can trap lightweight allergens such as cat dander that float in the air. (House dust mite material is too heavy and doesn't spend much time floating about. The allergens produced by pets are microscopic and are invisible to the naked eye.)
- Ban the pet from the main living rooms and bedrooms.
- Use the other methods listed for mites for carpets and furniture cleaning.
- Don't bother washing cats regularly – there is no convincing evidence that this helps. Cats are incredibly efficient at producing allergens – a weekly wash hardly puts them off their stride although they might decide to move out rather than put up with the treatment, so it could be an indirect solution! Washing a dog regularly might help reduce the amount of allergen on the animal but there will be still be plenty of it around the house.
- Un-neutered male cats produce more allergens than female cats, so consider a trip to the vet if you have a tom cat in the vicinity.

Moulds

It is impossible to avoid moulds and their spores completely as they are so widely spread throughout the air both indoors and outdoors. Measures to reduce mould indoors are the same as those for reducing humidity. Many people still seem to believe that modern houses are 'too dry' when in fact the reverse is usually the case. Older houses may be better ventilated if they are draughty but suffer from poorer insulation and condensation settles more easily in colder rooms. One therefore needs a compromise in which the house is kept reasonably warm but not excessively so, and air is allowed to circulate through open windows. This is not the most energy-efficient way of managing the home fuel bill, but turning down the heating by just a few degrees will cut most people's fuel consumption dramatically. Space heaters run on Calor gas should be avoided as they give off a lot of moisture and electric fan heaters kick up dust. Oil-filled electric space heaters are the most allergy-friendly and do not generate any moisture.

Moulds are particularly obvious in the dampest rooms, such as the kitchen and bathroom. Extractor fans can make a big difference to how long these take to clear of water vapour. Keeping the lids on boiling saucepans, avoiding drying clothes on indoor washing lines, wiping down showers and leaving an appropriate heater on in the bathroom are other common sense tips to reduce the humidity inside a house. New houses take ages to dry out and this is a process that can't be speeded up too much with de-humidifiers or else cracks will show up in the walls – open windows are the answer once again.

Pollens

Like moulds, pollens are unavoidable, although because they form heavier particles they do tend to settle more quickly indoors. The best you can do if you have a pollen allergy is to avoid going out on days with a high pollen count, avoid areas with lots of pollen such as meadowland and long grass, and don't have too many indoor plants. Pollen filters in cars might also be helpful but there is no scientific proof of this, and for them to work you need to leave all the windows shut. Antihistamine treatments have been the main help to pollen sufferers (chapter 5).

Exercise

Exercise is a common trigger for asthma attacks but the last thing anyone should do is avoid regular exercise solely on account of their asthma. Adequate asthma treatment should reduce symptoms enough to make exercise enjoyable again. However, jogging beside a main road is asking for trouble in the form of exhaust fumes and cycling beside fields at harvest time might not be sensible either. If you live in an inner city and don't have easy access to a park for walks you might have to compromise by timing a stroll for times of the day when there is less traffic on the roads. Try swimming, which is excellent exercise for all the muscles.

Drug therapy

Beta-blockers and aspirin sensitivity have already been mentioned as well-known triggers of asthma in some people, but there are other drugs that can cause asthma-type symptoms or which can clash with asthma medication. These interactions are not always spotted before they occur. For example, beta-blockers are also used in eye drops for a condition called glaucoma, but absorption of the drug in the eye drops can be sufficient to cause asthma. Should you have any concerns that your medicines are causing side effects you should always discuss this with your doctor.

Food allergy

This is an area that is particularly prone to be muddled by incorrect information. The first distinction to make is that between food allergy and food intolerance. Allergy to foods is similar to allergy to inhaled allergens in asthma. There is an interaction between the food and the immune system of the gut that triggers a response soon after the food is eaten. The close relationship in time makes it fairly easy to spot which foods cause the problem. Typical foods that can cause this are nuts, fish, shellfish and some fruits. It is unusual but not unknown for asthma to be triggered by foods in this way but generally the relationship is obvious and not in dispute.

The area of food intolerance is much more difficult. In this type of reaction some foods cause symptoms that occur hours or days later. It is much harder to prove a relationship between the food and the problems it causes, added to which is the concept that it could be foods that you have been used to eating for a long time that are responsible for the symptoms. Food intolerance is too near pseudo-science for many doctors, who therefore tend to dismiss it, but a less polarised view is preferable as there are occasional successes in people who have identified foods to which they are intolerant. The process of identification is lengthy and really beyond the scope of this book. Essentially it involves going on to a highly restricted diet for a while, during which time the symptoms of asthma (or other allergic condition such as eczema of the skin) will hopefully settle down. Then by slowly and successively introducing more variety into the diet one will identify the food that is associated with a return of the asthma symptoms. There is doubt over the scientific validity of these 'elimination' diets and all one can say is that they are an option for those who wish to explore every possible means of reducing their asthma symptoms and minimising their use of drug therapy. It is best to discuss with your doctor if you are going to try a highly restricted diet for a substantial period of time and to get advice from a qualified dietician.

Desensitisation

As we are discussing the subject of reducing the exposure to allergens it seems appropriate to mention the method of treatment called desensitisation, despite the fact that this has virtually disappeared from regular use in UK medical practice.

The principle behind desensitisation is similar to that of vaccination against infectious diseases. A small amount of a substance to which a person is allergic is repeatedly presented to the allergic person either as an injection under the skin or as drops under the tongue. The doses of the allergen are steadily increased until the person is able to tolerate them without the development of symptoms – in other words it is a method of building up tolerance to an allergen.

The reason this technique is so rarely done now in the UK dates back to 1986, when the Committee on Safety of Medicines (the regulatory body in the UK that oversees drug safety issues) recommended the withdrawal of the technique as there had been a small number of deaths associated with it. Perhaps this was an overly harsh ruling – desensitisation is still widely available in Europe and the USA – but people who wish to pursue this type of treatment in the UK will rarely if ever be able to get it via the NHS. Further studies are ongoing, however, to determine the true scientific value of this type of treatment, but as it stands it cannot be recommended.

SUMMARY

- Trigger factors for asthma should be identified where possible, first by experience and secondly by allergy tests in atopic individuals.
- Stopping smoking is essential for any asthmatic person.
- Sensible reduction of exposure to house dust mite includes mite-proofing of bedding materials and the removal or steam cleaning of carpets.
- Good ventilation and the avoidance of excess humidity reduce the build-up of mites and moulds within houses.
- Pet allergy is a significant cause of asthma.
- Occasionally drug therapy can cause or worsen asthma.
- Food allergy is rare but is usually easy to diagnose. Food intolerance is controversial and at best is a contributor to rather than a cause of asthma.
- Desensitisation therapy is essentially unavailable in the UK but is still being studied as a possible means of reducing the reaction to allergens.

Chapter 5

Treating Asthma (2) – Drug Therapy

Asthma is not curable but medication for asthma is now capable of considerably improving the quality of life of asthma sufferers, including those with very active disease. Because the site of action of the asthma process is within the bronchi, devices to deliver medicines to the airways have been developed, so in addition to the drugs themselves some consideration needs to be given to the different types of delivery device when looking at the way asthma treatment is used. Initially in this chapter an overview of the drugs is given, and in the second half of the chapter the main delivery devices are covered. More details of some specific drugs used in asthma treatment are in appendix B.

Steroids

The importance of the immune system and the process called inflammation in the development of asthma will now be clear. One of the most important aspects of modern asthma treatment is to reduce the inflammation within the bronchi, which improves the symptoms of asthma and reduces the long-term changes that can occur in the structure of the airways (airway remodelling). The most effective drugs for reducing inflammation, in all diseases including asthma, are steroids.

'Steroid' is a general term covering a large number of compounds with some similarities in structure. For example, the sex steroids are hormones produced by the testes in men and ovaries in women and which govern the sexual characteristics of men and women. The steroids that are concerned in the regulation of the inflammatory response originate in the adrenal glands, which are two walnut-sized pieces of tissue situated above each kidney. These compounds are referred to by the general term 'corticosteroids', or just 'steroids'. They are quite different from the steroids abused by misguided athletes.

Corticosteroids have been synthesised and manufactured artificially now for decades. When used as drug therapy the doses are much greater than the levels normally manufactured by the adrenal glands, and they have marked anti-inflammatory properties. Asthmatic people given steroid treatment show much less infiltration of their bronchi by the cells of the immune system, less bronchial narrowing and therefore more open airways. Steroids indirectly reduce the tendency of bronchial smooth muscle to contract, thus reducing the degree of spasm and narrowing of the airways. An asthmatic person treated with steroids will usually notice within a few days that they are less prone to attacks of wheeze, cough and breathlessness, especially at night and following exercise. Three steroids are in common use in the UK for inhalation treatment for asthma: beclometasone, budesonide and fluticasone. Beclometasone is the benchmark steroid and medical guidelines often refer to the dosage of this which is appropriate for the severity of the asthma.

SIDE EFFECTS OF STEROIDS

Side effects from inhaled steroids fall into two groups – those related to the local effects of the steroids that do not make it to the bronchi but instead get deposited in the throat and upper airways (which accounts for as much as 80 per cent of the inhaled dose) and those related to the absorption of the steroid into the body.

The main local effects are a mild weakening of the voice due to weakness of the muscles controlling the movement of the larynx ('voice box'). This is most noticeable in people who use their voice a lot at work. Spacer devices (see later) plus rinsing out the mouth after using the inhaler can reduce this problem. Thrush is an infection with yeasts that can be provoked by higher doses of inhaled steroids. It shows usually as a white patchy deposit at the back of the throat, or a generalised redness. Thrush is quite easy to treat with anti-fungal lozenges or gargles.

Absorption of steroids into the body gives rise to other side effects although the likelihood of such effects is much less than when steroids are taken by mouth. People who take high doses of inhaled steroids may show some tendency to bruising but there is no evidence that they suffer from weakening of the bones (osteoporosis) such as can occur with oral steroid use.

Of considerable concern has been whether the use of steroid inhalers in children can retard their growth. Conversely though it is known that poorly treated asthma itself causes a failure to grow properly. The consensus is that steroids for asthma in normal doses do not affect a child's growth, whereas high dose steroids may do, and these children (whose care is likely to need sharing with a specialist in childhood asthma) ought to have their growth monitored.

Sodium cromoglicate and nedocromil

These drugs are different from steroids but they also have anti-inflammatory properties. They stabilise various inflammatory cells such as the mast cells, preventing them from releasing histamine. Neither is of any use during an asthma attack – their value is to prevent asthma attacks occurring. They can be effective in reducing exercise-induced asthma: a single dose of sodium cromoglicate half an hour before exercise can prevent this. They may allow a reduction in the dose of inhaled steroids when taken along with this treatment.

Side effects from cromoglicate are almost unknown. The powder is a little heavy and can cause some throat irritation, but that's about all. Nedocromil can cause a bitter taste and headaches.

Leukotriene receptor antagonists

Leukotrienes are compounds released by immune system cells during asthma attacks and they are capable of causing bronchial smooth muscle to contract, thus narrowing the airways. Leukotriene receptor antagonists are relatively new drugs that block this effect, thus relaxing the airway muscle. There are two types available in the UK: montelukast, which can be used in all age groups down to two years old, and zafirlukast for people aged 12 and over. They can be used on their own or added to steroid treatment, where they may allow a reduction in steroid dose. Like cromoglicate they are effective in exercise-induced asthma but ineffective in an asthma attack. Side effects are uncommon and usually amount to digestive system upsets such as nausea but headaches and an unusual allergic condition involving the skin and blood vessels (called Churg-Strauss syndrome) have been reported.

Bronchodilators

These are drugs that relax the muscles of the bronchi, thus opening up the airways. The commonest of these are known by the term 'beta-2 agonists', or 'beta agonists', which refers to a technical aspect of their mode of action that is not important to know more about. Suffice to say that there are two types of beta-2 agonist: short-acting ones that work within minutes and last up to about four hours, and long-acting ones that work for about 12 hours after each dose. Beta-2 agonists work directly on the smooth muscle of the bronchioles and they do not have any anti-inflammatory powers.

The short-acting ones are salbutamol and terbutaline and the long-acting ones are salmeterol and formoterol. Short-acting bronchodilators are useful when a quick result is needed and long-acting drugs are good for night-time asthma attacks; however, the regular need for bronchodilators is an indication that someone's asthma is not under adequate control with anti-inflammatory drugs (such as steroids).

It is possible to give beta-2 agonists in oral form to young children who cannot use an inhaler properly but the effectiveness is low and the tendency to cause side effects is higher than with the inhaled drug. Side effects to beta-2 agonists are relatively few but they can include muscle shakes and a fast pulse.

The short-acting beta-2 agonists are the commonest drugs in use for the relief of asthma in the UK. Longer-acting beta-2 agonists are usually given alongside steroids and not on their own.

Theophylline

Theophylline has been around for decades and remains popular in many parts of the world. It is used as second-line treatment in the UK and is essentially a bronchodilator but may have weak anti-inflamma-tory properties too. It is given as slow-release tablets or capsules by mouth but can also be given by injection in emergencies (in a form called aminophylline). It is important not to give a theophylline injection to someone who is already taking oral theophylline as this may cause the blood level to become very high, which can cause disturbances of the heart rhythm or epileptic fits.

Provided the dose of theophylline is kept low enough then side effects are not serious but many people get headaches and digestive upset from theophylline. The slow-release forms tend to have fewer side effects and can be given once or twice a day. Ordinary (quick-release) tablets are still available but are less popular and need to be given three or four times daily. There are several proprietary forms of theophylline made by different manufacturers and people should stick to one brand so that they get consistent results. The pharmacist will check this happens if a brand is not specified on the doctor's prescription.

Anticholinergics

The name of this group of drugs comes from the general way in which they work. One of the controlling influences on the size of the airways is the nervous system. Nerves are distributed throughout lung tissue and are connected back to the spinal cord and brain (this is properly known as the autonomic nervous system). Like other automatic functions in the body such as blood pressure and temperature control, the activity of these nerves is not under our conscious control; nonetheless adjustments are made continuously to the bronchial muscles through the signals that pass through these nerves.

Anticholinergic drugs block these signals from getting through, thus causing the bronchial muscles to relax and the airways to open. They are less effective in this respect than beta-2 agonists but are useful medicines that can be used alongside other treatments. The two in common use are ipratropium and oxitropium. Tiotropium is a new anticholinergic and all of these drugs are more commonly used in chronic obstructive pulmonary disease (COPD – chapter 8). The side effects of anticholinergic drugs are minor and are caused through the blockage of cholinergic nerves elsewhere in the body (they are widely distributed). So a dry mouth and difficulty in passing urine can occur (the latter usually only in older men) and they can interfere with the eye condition called glaucoma if given via a nebuliser (see later in this chapter) so need to be avoided there.

Controllers and relievers

Two broad groups of asthma drug can be defined. **Controllers** (also called preventers) are those which dampen down the inflammation in asthmatic airways or which have a prolonged effect in keeping the airways open. These are:

- steroids
- sodium cromoglicate and nedocromil
- long-acting beta-2 agonists
- slow-release theophylline
- leukotriene receptor antagonists.

Relievers (also called rescue medication) are the drugs that can open up airways rapidly. These are:

- short-acting beta-2 agonists
- anticholinergics
- quick-release theophylline.

Antihistamines

As the name suggests, antihistamines are drugs that block the effect of histamine released by immune cells, which have been triggered by coming into contact with an allergen. Surprisingly they are ineffective in asthma but as asthma often co-exists with hay fever, for which they work well, they may end up being given for this reason in asthmatic people. Older antihistamines such as trimeprazine and promethazine tend to cause sedation. Chlorpheniramine is a commonly used antihistamine of the older type but is a bit less sedating. It can be purchased without a prescription. Modern antihistamines such as acrivastine, cetirizine and desloratadine cause little or no sedation. Ketotifen is an antihistamine that has been tried in asthma but with poor effect.

Inhaler devices

As asthma is a process involving the airways it is logical to deliver the treatment to the site of the problem. Inhaled treatments have the benefits of getting rapidly to where they are needed and of allowing the minimum amount of medication to be used to achieve the desired result. Thus beta-2 agonists can give relief within minutes of being inhaled and steroid inhalers largely avoid the general side effects of steroids that occur when they are taken by mouth. Not all drugs effective in asthma are suitable for inhaler delivery – leukotriene receptor antagonists and theophylline have to be given by mouth. There is now quite a large range of delivery devices made by different manufacturers, each with their own pros and cons. In general terms, one device is not 'better' than any other at achieving the aim of getting a dose of medicine into the airways, but there are differences in technique and convenience that can make some devices more suitable than others for a particular individual with asthma.

The choice of inhaler should be made with several aims in mind including ease of use, portability and personal preference on the part of the patient. Inhalers are not difficult to use – even for young children – but it is easy to misuse them one way or another. Inhaler technique is therefore something that is worth spending a bit of time on, and again this is one of the functions of the 'asthma nurse' who is increasingly often a member of the primary care team. Nurses trained in asthma care are also to be found in hospital clinics, and some of them also work in the community and can usefully bridge the gap, particularly where asthmatic children are concerned.

There are two main groups of inhaler device:

- pressurised 'metered dose' inhalers (MDI)
- dry powder inhalers.

Figure 6: Cross section of standard metered dose inhaler (MDI)

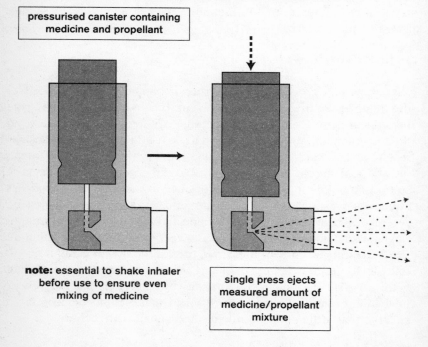

pressurised canister containing medicine and propellant

note: essential to shake inhaler before use to ensure even mixing of medicine

single press ejects measured amount of medicine/propellant mixture

PRESSURISED METERED DOSE INHALERS

These are the most familiar and are what most people think of when asked to describe an asthma inhaler. Figure 6 illustrates the general design.

A pressurised metal canister contains the active drug plus an inert propellant (gradually these are being changed over to environmentally-friendly propellants that do not contain CFCs). The canister is housed in a plastic holder and has a short exit tube that fits into a moulded spray channel. A single press down on the container ejects a precise amount of the drug, which is ejected through the spray channel, becoming an aerosol as it does so. By timing the intake of breath properly the patient catches the spray and carries it down into the lungs. Co-ordination of the puff with breathing in is important to maximise the efficiency of the inhaler. Self-triggering inhalers have a spring-loaded device above the canister that fires a dose when the patient breathes in, thus making the co-ordination automatic. They are slightly more bulky than the ordinary inhaler but are preferred by many people who find manual inhalers awkward to use. Otherwise they are no better than someone who can use an ordinary MDI well.

The elements of good inhaler technique are:

1. Sit up straight or stand up and lift the chin to open the airways.
2. Remove the cap from the mouthpiece and shake the inhaler vigorously.
3. If you haven't used the inhaler for a week or more, or it is the first time you have used the inhaler, spray it into the air first to check that it works.
4. Take a few deep breaths and then breathe out gently. Immediately place the mouthpiece in your mouth and put your teeth around it (not in front of it and do not bite it), and seal your lips around the mouthpiece, holding it between your lips.
5. Start to breathe in slowly and deeply through the mouthpiece. As you breathe in, simultaneously press down on the inhaler canister to release the medicine. One press releases one puff of medicine.
6. Continue to breathe in deeply to ensure the medicine gets into your lungs.

7. Hold your breath for 10 seconds or as long as you comfortably can, before breathing out slowly.
8. If you need to take another puff (2 puffs are commonly required for one dose), wait for 30 seconds, shake your inhaler again then repeat steps 4 to 7.
9. Replace the cap on the mouthpiece.

Practise using your inhaler in front of the mirror a few times. If you see mist coming from the top of the inhaler, or from the sides of your mouth, or your nostrils, you are not inhaling the dose correctly and the spray is escaping. If you can't get to grips with the co-ordination of an MDI, there are several other types of inhaler available (see below), so talk to your doctor, practice nurse or pharmacist for advice about which one may be best for you.

If you have weak hands you may find it easier to hold the inhaler with both hands and push the canister down with both index fingers rather than one. There is also a lever device available called a 'Haleraid', to help people use aerosol inhalers. Self-triggering inhalers are a better answer for those who have difficulty of this sort. It is important to clean an inhaler regularly about once a week, to prevent it getting clogged up. Remove the metal canister and mouthpiece cap from the case of the inhaler. Wash the case and cap in warm soapy water. Rinse in warm water then leave to dry. The holes in the valve sticking out of the bottom of the canister can sometimes become blocked – they can be cleaned with a pin if necessary but if you enlarge the hole the spray effect will be impaired. A blocked casing should be replaced as soon as possible.

Shaking the inhaler is important before dosing to ensure an even mix of the medicine and it also gives an idea of how much is left in the can. However, these miniature spray cans sometimes stop working before they are empty, which emphasises the need always to have a spare inhaler and not leave it too late before ordering your repeat prescription from your doctor. If an inhaler has packed up well before it should, return it to the pharmacist.

SPACERS

Although pressurised MDIs get the job done, they are inefficient. Even in people with good inhaler technique, only about 20 per cent of the drug actually reaches the lungs from each dose. The rest ends up on the inside of the mouth, the back of the throat and the upper airway. Mainly this is because the spray coming out of the inhaler is travelling at high speed in a more or less straight line. It then has to turn the corner at the back of the throat and negotiate the windpipe before it starts to get near to where it is needed.

Spacers are plastic attachments that improve the efficiency of inhalers. There are two main types (figure 7). Extension pieces simply increase the distance between the end of the inhaler and the patient's mouth. By the time the spray enters the mouth it is travelling more slowly, and evaporation has reduced the size of the droplets in the spray. Smaller droplets can turn corners more easily, so less medicine ends up on the sides of the upper airway and throat. These spacers still require proper co-ordination between pressing the inhaler and breathing in at the right time.

Chamber spacers are larger and are designed to trap a dose of the aerosol within a sealed plastic bubble which has a valve at the mouthpiece. One puff of the medicine is fired into the chamber and then one can take a few normal breaths through the mouthpiece, which gets the medicine into the lungs without the need for any co-ordination. Chamber spacers are bulkier than the extension type, but are suitable for anyone, including children. Masks are available for young children.

Plastic chamber spacers tend to become charged with static electricity, which attracts particles of the medicine and makes them stick to the chamber, where they can't help the patient! Static can be eliminated by rinsing the spacer in a detergent solution and letting it dry naturally (drying with a cloth re-charges the spacer with static). Different manufacturers make different spacers and some fit only one make, whereas others can be used with several makes. They are all available on prescription. Once you've found a combination that suits you, then stick with it.

Figure 7: 'Spacer' devices

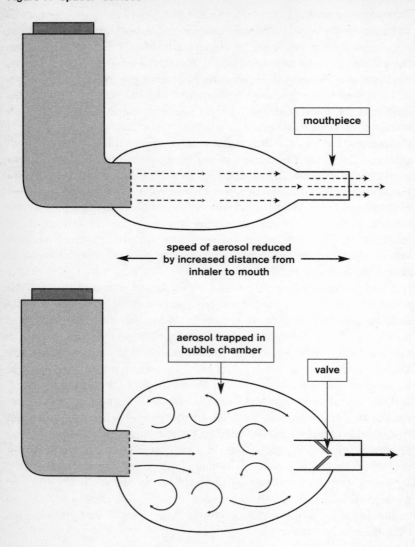

speed of aerosol reduced
by increased distance from
inhaler to mouth

DRY POWDER INHALERS

This is the other main type of inhaler. They do not use propellants and rely only on a sharp intake of breath to work. Co-ordination problems are therefore less than with pressurised MDIs. Several types of dry powder inhaler (DPI) are in use. The original, and still widely used, type has each dose in a plastic capsule, which is punctured and spun as the patient breathes in. More recent variations on this theme use blister packs, each blister containing a dose of drug. These types all bulk out the dose with a small amount of finely ground lactose (sugar) to make the dispersal of the drug run more efficiently. The Turbohaler® device delivers the pure drug each time, so the amount of powder in each dose is very small and tasteless. These look like pepper pots and are charged for use by a twist of the base. Blister devices and Turbohalers have indicators to show how many doses are left. In the case of the Turbohaler this takes the form of a window on the side of the device that shows red when 10 or fewer doses remain. (Shaking a Turbohaler gives a noise, which is due to the internal moisture-absorbing material and has nothing to do with how much is left in it.)

Dry powder inhalers are equal to or are better than pressurised MDIs in efficiency. Turbohalers can deliver twice as much medicine to the airways if the intake of air is fast enough. This doesn't necessarily mean they achieve better asthma control – the best inhaler to use is the one that you get on with. They are all capable of treating asthma well.

Side effects from DPIs are similar to those of the pressurised variety and are due to the medicine landing up on the back of the throat or on the vocal cords. Thrush (yeast) infection is fairly common with high dose steroid treatment, as it is with aerosols. Rinsing and gargling after using the inhaler minimises throat irritation. Spacers are of course unnecessary with dry powder inhalers.

NEBULISERS

Nebulisers are powered devices that create a fine mist of an asthma drug, which can be breathed in over a period of a few minutes to deliver a reasonably high amount of drug to the airways. They are particularly useful in more severe asthma attacks and in children and adults who find it hard to use inhalers. The simplest and commonest types have a small air pump that delivers a steady supply of air to a plastic chamber containing the medicine in liquid form. The chamber is designed to create a mist of the medicine, which is breathed in either through a face-mask or, more effectively, through a plastic mouthpiece. It takes a few minutes for each dose to run through, during which time it is necessary only to take normal breaths. More expensive nebulisers use ultrasound to create the mist. Their only real advantage is that they run quietly, whereas the air-powered devices can be a bit noisy.

SUMMARY
- 'Controller' medicines for asthma reduce inflammation in the airways and/or have a long-acting effect of keeping airways open. They are: steroids, sodium cromoglicate/nedocromil, long-acting beta-2 agonists, slow-release theophylline and leukotriene receptor antagonists.
- Relievers act quickly to relieve bronchospasm. They are: short-acting beta-2 agonists, anticholinergics and quick-release theophylline.
- Steroids are the mainstay of therapy to reduce inflammation of the airways in asthma.
- The side effects of inhaled steroids are generally very low and they can be safely used in all age groups.
- Pressurised metered dose inhalers are the commonest type, but also the hardest to use correctly.
- Spacers improve the efficiency of pressurised inhalers.
- Dry powder inhalers require less co-ordination and are potentially more efficient than aerosol types.
- The best type of inhaler needs to be decided on an individual basis.
- Nebulisers are powered devices that can deliver a steady flow of asthma medication and are useful in more severe asthma attacks, or in people who find other inhalers hard to use.

Chapter 6

Managing Asthma – Stepwise Treatment

Much of the information in this book is derived from the recommendations of the Global Initiative for Asthma (GINA) – a worldwide network of asthma and public health experts and organisations whose purpose is to ensure that the best information about asthma management reaches the patients through those who care for them.

The goals of asthma treatment set out by GINA are to:

- achieve and maintain control of symptoms
- prevent asthma exacerbations
- maintain lung function as close to normal as possible
- maintain normal activity levels, including exercise
- avoid adverse effects from asthma medications
- prevent development of irreversible airflow restriction
- prevent deaths from asthma.

People with asthma need information about the condition that they understand and can act upon, and it is the aim of this book to contribute to that goal. They also need guidance from their carer – be it doctor or nurse – on how to manage their asthma, because everyone is different. General principles, however, can be applied and much effort in recent years has gone into establishing what these principles should be. The outcome has been a 'step approach' to asthma care, which is widely accepted across the world.

The steps in question are based on the severity of someone's asthma, and there are four of them. Ideally each asthmatic person should know the essentials about what step they are on, and what to do about it should their asthma go one way or the other. A management plan is therefore required for everyone with asthma, and it should be the goal of the health care services to ensure this happens. For example this might set out under what circumstances it would be right for a person with asthma to start on a home supply of oral steroid tablets should their asthma begin to deteriorate over a short period of time. This might prevent the attack from getting worse but there would also be clear guidelines on when to call for assistance from the doctor if improvement was slow or inadequate. Self management plans encourage the patient's independence without sacrificing safety and are increasingly part of good asthma management.

What follows covers the main points of the step approach to asthma care, but it is not intended as a management plan for anyone. That can only be done on an individual basis and worked out between you and your doctor and asthma nurse.

As the step system is based on asthma severity one needs a way of measuring severity. This is done in a simple way by assessing the symptoms experienced and taking into account the peak flow reading, compared with the expected best reading for the individual patient. This will become clearer as we go through the steps. Underpinning all of the steps is the need to minimise exposure to allergens and to be competent at using and sticking to one's prescribed medication.

Step 1

This is intermittent asthma, in which there is less than a daily need for one dose of a beta-2 agonist reliever. Night-time asthma symptoms occur less than twice a month, there are no symptoms between exacerbations and PEFR is normal (80 per cent or more of predicted best). Controller medicine is not required on this step.

Step 2

This is the 'mild persistent' level. Patients will wake at night with a cough or wheeze, but less often than once a week. They may need daily reliever medication. Their average peak flow is normal but they show 20–30 per cent variability in the readings during or between days.

On step 2 one needs to be on a daily dose of a controller medicine. Most doctors prefer a steroid as first choice but one could try sodium cromoglicate or nedocromil in children. Some doctors will try a leuko-triene receptor antagonist instead but this is less well established as a choice.

Step 3

'Moderate persistent' symptoms occur daily over many weeks, or occur at night more than once a week. PEFR is 60–80 per cent at baseline and varies by more than 30 per cent. As with all the steps, one needs to continue using short-acting beta-2 inhalers as required for quick relief but also to use higher doses of inhaled steroid to which one can add a long-acting bronchodilator. This can be particularly helpful for night-time symptoms. Any deterioration from this level, i.e. a need for reliever medicine more often than four-hourly, or unrelieved breath-lessness, will probably require a course of oral steroids and a doctor's advice should be obtained without delay.

Step 4

At this level symptoms are continuous, sleep is frequently disturbed, activities are limited and exacerbations are severe despite treatment.

Medication comprises regular short-acting beta-2 inhalers, high dose inhaled steroids and a sequential trial of one or more of:

- inhaled long-acting beta-2 inhaler
- slow-release theophylline
- anticholinergic inhaler
- long-acting beta-2 agonist tablets
- high-dose inhaled bronchodilator
- sodium cromoglicate or nedocromil.

Many specialists add step 5, which is essentially step 4 plus the addition of regular daily steroid tablets. Patients on step 5 will also be on high dose inhaled steroids.

Stepping down

Every three to six months one should ideally review asthma treatment, particularly for those people taking a lot of medication. If there has been an improvement and this has been stable for a while then a drop in treatment can be tried. The aim is always to achieve the best control of asthma with the minimum amount of side effects but too much chopping and changing may be counterproductive if the asthma becomes unstable.

Severe asthma

No one with asthma, even if it has been mild for a long time, is free from the risk of getting a severe attack. The numbers of people dying from asthma have fortunately been falling for several years but the numbers of people being admitted to hospital with severe attacks has not fallen. In 75 per cent or more cases of fatal asthma attacks there is evidence that earlier action could have saved that person's life. Everyone therefore needs to know how to recognise severe asthma, and what to do about it.

The severity of an asthma attack is judged by its effects at the time, not by how long it has been going on. Among the many risk factors that increase the chance of severe attacks is the fact that some people just put up with severe symptoms for hours, days or even weeks before seeking help, or being forced to get it.

A severe attack is present if:

- PEFR is less than 50 per cent of predicted best.
- One is too breathless to complete a sentence.
- Breathing rate is 25 breaths a minute or greater.
- Pulse rate is 110 beats per minute or greater.

These are just guides and you can be in trouble from asthma without showing any of these features. If in doubt, always ask a doctor. The correct treatment of a severe asthma attack is to dial 999. It is not a DIY condition. While waiting for the ambulance to come, sit down and take as much control of your breathing as you can. There can be a large amount of understandable anxiety in an asthma attack, which can cause you to breathe too quickly (hyperventilate). This sets off another chain of events in the body that can make you feel very faint or develop pins and needles in your hands and feet. Bringing down the rate of breathing controls this. In no circumstances try breathing into a bag for this symptom – you need all the oxygen you can get. Although it is likely that you will have been using your reliever medication a lot in an attempt to improve your breathing, check that the inhaler is actually working. If in doubt, open up the spare. Use a spacer if you have one to improve the penetration of the medicine into the bronchi. A chamber spacer can be used as a makeshift nebuliser by charging it with extra doses of reliever – but this is only meant to be a temporary measure until professional help arrives.

Of course one wants to steer away from getting a bad attack, so seek help if you notice:

- an increasing need for reliever medication
- a fall in PEFR, especially if over a short period of time

77

- worsening of cough, wheeze, breathlessness
- new symptoms such as night wakening if you didn't have this before.

Although these are all signs that your asthma is not well controlled they do not automatically mean you are heading for a severe attack. But if you get your treatment sorted out at this stage you may never get any worse. The PEFR can be very helpful in gauging how 'tight' your asthma is, and it is worth getting in the habit of using it. If you have ever had a severe asthma attack in the past you are at increased risk of having one again, so have an even lower threshold for seeking advice if your asthma begins to deteriorate.

Anaphylaxis

The most extreme form of allergic reaction is anaphylaxis (anaphylactic shock) – a potentially life-threatening event caused by someone coming into contact with an allergen to which they are extremely sensitive. Like atopic asthma, anaphylaxis is usually triggered through IgE combining with the allergen and then leading to the release of substances like histamine into the bloodstream, but this time in very much larger amounts. Anaphylactic reactions are more likely in atopic people but can occur in anyone. The commonest allergens to trigger such a reaction are insect stings, injected drugs or vaccinations, as these get into the body tissues. Less commonly the oral intake of shellfish, nuts or other food or drugs can cause anaphylaxis.

The symptoms include an itchy rash, wheeze, abdominal cramps, swelling of the tongue or throat, breathlessness and fainting. Not all of these might occur and a full blown anaphylactic reaction is rare. First aid treatment is to keep the person on their side if they have collapsed and call for assistance right away. It can become necessary to use resuscitation (CPR) in the worst cases – first aid training in how to carry out CPR is widely available and everyone should learn this skill.

Someone with a potential to get severe allergic reactions should discuss with their doctor whether they should carry an adrenaline-loaded syringe. These are specially designed for emergency use. Adrenaline can rapidly reverse an anaphylactic reaction. They should also see a specialist in allergic diseases both for advice and to try and accurately identify the allergen.

SUMMARY

- Basic asthma treatment measures, such as reducing the exposure to irritants, having good inhaler technique and complying with prescribed treatment, apply to everyone.
- Taking into account symptoms and measures such as the peak flow rate allows a simple grading of asthma severity, upon which to base 'steps' of asthma treatment.
- Each asthmatic person should have an individual asthma management plan, worked out in conjunction with their doctor or nurse, which indicates what changes to look for in their symptoms, and what to do about them.
- Severe asthma attacks can occur in anyone but are usually preceded by warning signs. If these are recognised and acted upon in time, many fewer people would get such attacks.
- If in doubt, always ask.

Chapter 7

Asthma in Children

Many of the points relating to the occurrence of asthma in childhood have already been made. Wheeze is common in infants and asthma is commoner in children than in adults. A significant minority of asthmatic children carry their condition into adulthood but most do not. Most wheezy infants have stopped wheezing by the time they get to primary school.

Although the basic principles of asthma treatment are the same in children as they are for adults, there are important differences. Parents can be understandably reluctant to accept a diagnosis of asthma in childhood, and often it is impossible to make a dogmatic statement that a child is or is not asthmatic. 'Cough-variant asthma' is probably over-diagnosed in children who go on coughing for a long time following upper airway infections but who are not really asthmatic.

It's better not to get too worked up about diagnostic labels in this age group, but to take a more practical stance. Children who have asthma-type symptoms will be likely to respond to asthma-type treatment. They might need that for some months or even years – time will tell. If in the meantime a sensible approach is taken to using the least amount of medicine that keeps them free of symptoms then that's what really matters. Every now and again one can try to withdraw the medication completely if there have been no symptoms for a while. Provided one uses some common sense and restarts treatment if symptoms begin to recur then no harm has been done.

What is most important is that a good diagnosis is made in the first place, i.e. a look for other causes of the same symptoms is carried out – the younger the child the more alternative possibilities there are that can cause similar symptoms. These include fairly common problems such as the reflux of stomach acid that spills over into the top of the windpipe, to rarities of development of the muscles or nerves of the throat – the list is a long one.

Treating very young children for asthma is problematic because it is so difficult to get medication to them effectively. Young children can get the hang of a chamber spacer with a kiddies' mask attachment but children below two really don't like them. For a mask/spacer combination to work it has to be applied to the child's face so that a gas seal is achieved – holding the mask near the face doesn't work.

Oral medications containing bronchodilators are better than nothing but not by much and as soon as possible a child who needs asthma medication needs inhaled treatment. There is a temptation to use a nebuliser to achieve this. Although fine for acute attacks nebulisers are very inconvenient for regular drug dosing, and there is no evidence that they are better at delivering drugs to the airways than inhalers.

Although adult asthma has been much researched and care methods have been well worked out, the same is not true of childhood asthma, which is difficult to research, difficult to diagnose and difficult to treat. The stepped approach to asthma management is really an adult-oriented scheme and its application to children is mainly because we don't have a better scheme to go by that's been tailored to the needs of young people. This doesn't necessarily mean that following the same general guidance for children will be wrong, but it is not based on a strong scientific basis.

Where there is doubt about the diagnosis or a need for help in treating an infant or child with asthma, help should be sought from a consultant with a special interest in the condition.

Chapter 8

Chronic Obstructive Pulmonary Disease

Chronic obstructive pulmonary disease, or COPD, is a general term for several lung conditions that also cause restriction of airflow, breathlessness and wheeze. COPD is not asthma, but it is often confused with asthma and has several similarities to it. The primary difference in definition between the two conditions is that in asthma the airways obstruction is partially or largely reversible whereas in COPD it is not, but in real life this distinction is not so clear-cut. In fact distinguishing COPD from longstanding asthma can be very difficult indeed, especially in people who have smoked.

COPD occurs mainly in smokers or ex-smokers, and those who have smoked most and for the longest have the greatest risk of lung damage. However, the lung changes of COPD do not affect all smokers – only 10–20 per cent seem to develop it, indicating that there are other factors involved. As we don't know much about what those other factors are, every smoker in effect takes a gamble on developing

COPD, amongst all the other problems that smoking causes.

Microscopic study of the lung tissue in COPD shows invasion by inflammatory cells, much like asthma, but other changes that are different. A form of scarring develops in COPD as well as a breakdown of the structure of the alveoli, which is properly called emphysema. In advanced emphysema whole sections of lung tissue have damaged alveoli, greatly reducing their ability to absorb oxygen and get rid of carbon dioxide.

Diagnosis

By the time most people with COPD come to the doctor about it they are already getting breathless and wheezy, and have usually lost a good deal of their lung function already. They will almost certainly also have a history of longstanding cough, but will probably have just put up with that for years and blamed it on the cigarette smoking.

Someone with established COPD tends to have a characteristically barrel-shaped chest – as if they are permanently holding in a deep breath. Wheeze, usually worse on breathing out, is due to a combination of spasm of the bronchi as well as 'air trapping' by damaged alveoli, which collapse on breathing out, blocking the exit of air from neighbouring alveoli. Someone with advanced COPD learns by experience to breathe out through pursed lips, which keeps the pressure in the airways higher than normal. In turn this keeps the alveoli from collapsing and actually makes it easier to exhale.

Lung function tests of a slightly more complex type than the basic peak flow reading show a pattern which indicates COPD, and the next step is to find out if there is any 'reversibility' to it. This can be done by measuring lung function before and after a bronchodilator or following a course of a few weeks' steroid treatment by inhaler or by mouth. Most people with COPD show some improvement on either therapy.

Treatment

Until fairly recently many doctors looked upon COPD as an untreatable disease – the definition of irreversible airways obstruction did nothing to discourage that belief. Perhaps because so many sufferers were also smokers a little bit of moralising crept into that attitude too. However, the modern view of COPD is not so negative.

Stopping smoking is the top priority and stops the decline in lung function that otherwise goes on relentlessly. It really is never too late to stop.

Bronchodilator treatments (beta-2 agonists and anticholinergics) are the main treatments that help. Because of the type of lung damage in COPD small improvements in airway size can give quite good symptom improvement – more than the equivalent in asthma. The type of inhaler can matter a lot in COPD as many patients find them difficult to use, in which case a nebuliser is a better option.

The use of steroid inhalers in COPD used to be advised only for those people who showed an improvement in their lung function tests after a trial period on the drugs but this is an area that is being looked at again. Some patients who remain on steroids get fewer exacerbations and perhaps have slower rates of lung deterioration. As yet it is not possible to pick out those who would benefit most but usually people with severe COPD are offered regular inhaled steroid treatment just in case. Oral steroids, however, are of no long-term value in COPD and can be a disadvantage, adding to the muscle weakness that often accompanies advanced COPD. Short courses of oral steroids may, however, be necessary for exacerbations.

Infections can be a major setback. If possible people with colds should keep away from anyone with COPD and usually antibiotics will be needed if an infection is caught. Influenza vaccine is generally routine for COPD sufferers.

Oxygen therapy

Advanced lung damage can make it so difficult to get about that oxygen therapy becomes an option, although this will still mean that the person is housebound. Oxygen can be provided either in cylinders, which are heavy, awkward to move about and need frequent replacement, or by a 'concentrator' – a machine about the size of a bedside cabinet that provides an enriched oxygen supply from the air. Oxygen treatment is of proven benefit only for people with very low blood oxygen levels breathing air. It needs to be used for at least 15 hours a day and the patient is restricted in moving around by the length of the tubing. A specialist in chest medicine needs to decide when it will be beneficial.

Surgery

In carefully selected patients surgery to the lungs can be helpful. For example, some people develop large air-filled sacs in the lungs due to a merging of damaged alveoli. Removal of these can let the rest of the lung operate more effectively. Other forms of surgery all the way up to lung transplantation are feasible, although applicable to only a small proportion of COPD sufferers.

COPD is a serious condition and is not curable, but it can be helped. People with COPD should be seen by a specialist in chest medicine, who can advise on the best treatment at all stages of the illness, but only those patients who give up smoking will experience any real benefit from treatment.

Chapter 9

Complementary Treatments for Asthma

One of the biggest growth areas in recent years has been in complementary medicine. The reasons are not hard to find as people increasingly feel disinclined to take medications on a long-term, or even short-term, basis. There is a lot of appeal in trying to 'get to the cause' of a problem rather than trying to mask it, as the conventional medical approach is often perceived to do, although complementary treatments rarely achieve that goal either. Drugs have side effects, some of them serious, and one tends to hear more about those in the media than about the success stories, which are usually less sensational. Although many doctors remain dismissive of complementary treatments more now see them as worthy of some place in an overall scheme of medicine, which acknowledges that no one has all the answers. The duty that conventional medicine has is to offer an objective view of the evidence for and against these treatments, and let the individual decide if he or she wishes to use them.

Asthma is a popular area for experimentation in complementary treatments – one survey of 4741 UK asthma sufferers showed that 59 per cent of them had tried one or other form of it for their condition.

The pros and cons of specific complementary treatments for asthma are discussed below with reference to randomised controlled trials (RCTs). An RCT is a study in which people are allocated at random to receive one of several clinical 'interventions' – usually a drug but it could be any other type of treatment such as physiotherapy, counselling, massage and so on. Another intervention is regarded as the standard of comparison, or control. The control might be another type of pre-existing treatment whose effectiveness is known or it could be a placebo. Placebos are most commonly used in drug trials, and look, taste and feel the same as the active treatment. The 'placebo effect', in which someone feels better taking *any* treatment, including an 'inactive' one, exists in asthma just as much as in most other medical conditions.

It is much more difficult to conduct a placebo-controlled trial when the intervention under test is something as obvious as acupuncture, for example – it is pretty hard to convince someone that they are getting a needle stuck into them when they are not! However, such limitations have to be accepted in testing many forms of complementary treatment and a compromise reached in doing a fair comparison with conventional treatment. In the case of acupuncture, for example, the control group usually receives 'sham' treatment in which the needles are put into points which are not recognised acupuncture positions. Usually RCTs seek to measure and compare different events that are present or absent after the participants in the study receive the interventions. These events are called outcomes.

Acupuncture

A systematic review looking at the use of complementary medicine in the treatment of asthma and asthma-like symptoms assessed seven acupuncture studies. Two of these studies suggested that real acupuncture was superior to sham acupuncture. The other five studies found no significant advantage and the authors therefore concluded that, 'it is not yet possible to make any recommendations'.

When properly done acupuncture is a safe treatment. It probably has a large and clinically relevant 'placebo effect' because it is often associated with great expectations and so the pros and cons depend mostly on an individual's opinion. Someone who considers only evidence from trials would not advocate the use of acupuncture, whereas someone with a more practical clinical stance might believe that it is worth trying, if only for its placebo effect.

Homoeopathy

A systematic review of all RCTs on homoeopathy in asthma included only three studies. Two of them suggested a benefit beyond placebo on at least one outcome measure. The authors concluded that the evidence was insufficient to assess the possible role of homoeopathy in the treatment of asthma. Weighing the pros and cons of homoeopathy for asthma, one therefore arrives at much the same conclusions as for acupuncture.

Exclusion diets

About 2 to 6 per cent of asthma sufferers are hypersensitive to foods and experience worsening symptoms when they eat certain foods. It is reasonable, therefore, for these individuals to exclude the offending foodstuff from their diet. Curiously, the effectiveness of this approach has not been clearly confirmed through RCTs. On balance, it seems that this technique is worth trying in patients for whom hypersensitivity to foods has been established.

Other nutritional approaches

The role of vitamins, minerals and essential fatty acids in the management of asthma remains unclear. There are some data that suggest that the addition of such nutrients could have a positive effect. However, not enough trials have been done. As a result there is, at present, no compelling evidence that other nutritional approaches are effective in the treatment or prevention of asthma.

Breathing techniques

Many breathing techniques (including yoga) are promoted for alleviating the symptoms of asthma. A systematic review of all the available trial evidence found some promising, albeit not compelling, evidence for yoga and conventional physiotherapeutic techniques. Moreover, there is some (again, not compelling) evidence to suggest that the Buteyko technique is of some benefit. This technique, developed over 50 years ago by the Russian scientist Konstantin Pavlovich Buteyko, is a set of simple breathing exercises to encourage shallow breathing. Buteyko breathing does not improve asthma but it can help improper breathing that might accompany asthma in some people. On balance, therefore, it is worth trying with adequate supervision.

Hypnosis

Hardly any RCTs have tested the effectiveness of hypnosis for asthma. Two small trials yielded encouraging results but it is unclear to what extent this benefit was due to placebo effects. Nonetheless, the balance of the evidence seems positive and so hypnosis, under adequate medical supervision, seems to be worth trying for suitable patients, who might be those in whom stress and anxiety are significant accompanying problems.

Relaxation techniques

A systematic review of all RCTs on this topic had mixed results. Two studies showed no benefit while another two did suggest improvement. A further two studies demonstrated statistically significant but clinically irrelevant effects. One trial of Jacobsonian relaxation (a technique in which relaxation is learnt by tensing and relaxing skeletal muscle) in boys was followed by clinical improvement. In view of the overall safety of relaxation therapy and at least some indication that it is beneficial, relaxation techniques seem to be worth trying.

Chiropractic

Perhaps surprisingly, chiropractic is often promoted for asthma. The concept is that spinal manipulation could improve lung function by freeing restrictions of rib movements and reducing muscle tension. Two RCTs, however, clearly showed that chiropractic is not useful beyond a placebo effect for asthma.

Herbal medicine

A systematic review has found 17 RCTs of herbal medicinal products for asthma. The overall quality of the trials was poor. Six studies concerned the use of traditional Chinese medicine, four of which reported a clinically significant increase in FEV1 of 15 per cent or more (FEV1 is the forced expiratory volume in one second – a measure of lung function). However, it is difficult to interpret the validity of trials of traditional Chinese medicine because of:

- inadequate trial methods
- lack of standardisation of dosages of active ingredients (e.g. ephedrine)
- different classifications of asthma used
- lack of reports of adverse effects, patient drop-out or withdrawal rates.

Five RCTs investigated the use in asthma of *Tylophora indica*, a perennial climbing plant native to Southern and Eastern India, where it is a traditional remedy for asthma and hay fever. The evidence was inconclusive, with three of the studies reporting very significant benefits and two (more recent) trials finding no improvement at all. Other traditional medicines that have been tested include *Picrorhiza kurroa* (roots of a Himalayan herb), *Solanum species* (potato family), *Boswellia serrata* (frankincense), *Saiboku-to* (Japanese herb), marijuana and dried ivy extract. In all cases, the evidence was inconclusive. The bottom line therefore is that herbal remedies cannot be recommended for the treatment of asthma.

Massage

Massage is calming and potentially beneficial for asthma, but has rarely been investigated for this condition. In one recent study, children were randomised to receive 20 minutes of either massage or relaxation instruction from their parents. Children aged six to eight years who received massage had improvements in short-term anxiety and lung function at 30 days, which was significantly better than the relaxation controls. In the older children aged nine to 11 years, there was no significant difference between the two treatment groups. Thus the role of massage therapy in the treatment of asthma seems to be minor.

Conclusion

Even though some complementary therapies show promise and deserve to be investigated in more detail, at present there is no compelling evidence to show that any such treatment does more good than harm in the treatment of asthma. None could be said to be positively harmful, unless of course they encouraged someone to stop the asthma treatment that they needed or otherwise adversely affected their conventional treatment. As most have a positive effect on well-being they should be seen to be possibly useful treatments from that point of view. Unfortunately almost no complementary treatments are available via the NHS. There are professional organisations for some of these therapies that can provide the names of qualified practitioners.

Chapter 10

Asthma in Special Circumstances

Pregnancy

Having asthma should pose no problems to giving birth to a healthy baby but often asthmatic mothers experience a change in their level of symptoms during the pregnancy. It's said that about a third get better, a third get worse and a third stay the same. The risk of an exacerbation of asthma is highest just after the baby is born but quite rapidly the asthma will settle to its usual level. Often the pattern of an individual woman's asthma is the same in subsequent pregnancies.

None of the medicines commonly used in asthma have shown any special risk to a developing baby, although the experience with newer medicines such as the leukotriene antagonists is necessarily less than for drugs like salbutamol which have been around for decades.

What is clear is that poorly controlled asthma poses a much greater risk to the baby (and the mother) than any worry over drug side effects. Babies born to mothers whose asthma is out of control are more likely to be premature, small, and to have an increased risk of dying at or around birth. The converse is also true, i.e. babies born to mothers whose asthma is well controlled are as likely to be healthy as those from non-asthmatic mothers.

Good asthma treatment and monitoring is therefore to be sought after, and can best be done by planning ahead, even before conception. It is a good idea for prospective mums to discuss in advance with their GP, midwife, health visitor or asthma nurse any worries they have about the possible effects of their treatment on the baby. As always the aim of treatment is to get control of the asthma using the least amount of medicine, but it is safer to err on the side of slightly too much than too little in this condition. The main message should, however, be quite clear: asthma and pregnancy can and do co-exist perfectly well.

Operations and anaesthetics

One of the many jobs of an anaesthetist is to ensure that when someone needs an anaesthetic they get the safest type that allows the surgeon to carry out the operation properly. Procedures on the lower half of the body and legs can therefore often be done using injections which 'freeze' the nerves there but which allow the patient to remain awake (epidural or spinal injections). From the chest point of view this is the best option, with the least risk of lung complications afterwards.

For many types of operation, however, there is no alternative to a general anaesthetic. Usually these also involve the need for a breathing tube to be placed into the trachea during the operation. People with chest trouble of any sort, including asthma, are at a higher risk of complications from such anaesthetics, but this can be minimised by ensuring the asthma is under good control well in advance of going into hospital. Therefore a review of symptom control a few weeks ahead is a good idea, especially for people with more troublesome asthma. The anaesthetist may also suggest extra measures such as a short course of steroid tablets for a few days before the operation to dampen down any inflammation in the airways. Any signs of infection such as increased cough, breathlessness, dirty spit or a temperature will almost always mean that the operation is best postponed to another day unless it is an emergency (this applies to everyone, not just those with asthma). Applying common sense rules such as this ensures that the vast majority of people with asthma who undergo surgery do so just as safely as anyone else.

Asthma and sport

We all need to exercise regularly to keep healthy and enjoy life for longer. Having asthma is no bar to exercise, and many world-class athletes and sportspersons are asthmatic. Exercise is, however, a common trigger factor for asthma, and in some people is the single most important one. Often this is referred to as 'exercise-induced asthma', or EIA.

Using a peak flow meter before and after a vigorous burst of exercise may show the characteristic drop in the reading of 20–30 per cent or more but often the asthmatic person's symptoms are a giveaway that they need more treatment. Typically a young person will not last a game of football without needing to stop for breath or to cough, or they'll be particularly fatigued by running about. Sometimes this is how asthma first shows itself, especially in active teenagers.

Any form of exercise can potentially trigger asthma but some are more prone to do so than others. Long-distance running requires sustained periods of increased demand on the lungs and is more likely than sprinting to be accompanied by EIA. Running on cold days is worse as the cold air does not have time to warm up in its passage through the nose and upper airway, whereas swimming is usually good exercise in asthma as the air from the pool is warm and moist, and so is less irritating to the airways. (The exception here is if someone's asthma is particularly sensitive to chlorine in the pool water.)

Exercise-induced symptoms can mean that someone's asthma is under-treated. This might mean there is a need to move up a step in treatment, as described in chapter 6, but if the symptoms are very much limited to sports activity it may be enough just to take an extra couple of puffs of a quick-acting bronchodilator like salbutamol to get you through a football game, for example. Other strategies might need to be worked out on an individual basis, such as the use of cromoglicate or nedocromil prior to a race, or using a long-acting bronchodilator or leukotriene antagonist temporarily if these are not justified to be used regularly. Exercise-induced asthma can be a particular challenge in children who are very sporty and trying for competitive success but there is usually an answer to be found, even if it needs a bit of experimentation to find it. Some doctors have a special interest in sports medicine and asthma, and usually your GP will know who that is and can refer you or your child if necessary.

Asthma medication and sport

Exercise is of course for everyone, not just the tiny number of elite athletes but for those who are engaged in competitive sport the issue of medication for asthma is one that has been well covered by the relevant governing bodies. In brief, all inhaled medications and most oral medications required for the necessary treatment of asthma are allowed substances. The use of some (such as salbutamol and terbutaline, i.e. quick-acting bronchodilators) are in the restricted category, which means that you need written confirmation from a doctor that you need the medication. Others, such as leukotriene antagonists and theophylline, have no restrictions in their use. A full database of drugs and their status in sport is available on the UK Sport web site at www.uksport.gov.uk.

Scuba diving

There is little or no firm evidence that someone with mild or well-controlled asthma is at any higher risk than the non-asthmatic person who does scuba diving. Nonetheless some countries still impose an absolute ban on this activity by asthmatic people. The UK advice is more liberal, and can be accessed on the British Sub Aqua Club's web site at http://www.bsac.org. This states that someone should not dive if they have needed a bronchodilator (to relieve wheeze) in the preceding 48 hours, although it is acceptable (and a good idea) to take a dose prior to diving as a preventative measure. People should not dive if they have asthma which is triggered by exercise, cold or emotion. These restrictions would cover a very high proportion of people with asthma, but well-controlled asthmatics may dive, so there is clearly some room for interpretation of the medical criteria. This should be done by a doctor recognised by the BSAC. The rules are there for safety's sake although it may disappoint someone with troublesome asthma who is keen to dive to know that they would be disallowed.

Mountaineering and skiing

Living at high altitude is generally good for asthma because of the reduced levels of pollutants and allergens in the air, although at very high altitudes the reduced oxygen levels and temperature of the air act as aggravating factors. Even those who live above the pollution may still have a high incidence of asthma related to house dust mite or animal dander in their homes.

Other lung problems such as pulmonary oedema (fluid in the lungs) occur in a small proportion of all people who ascend rapidly to high altitude and this is unrelated to the presence of asthma. In the case of lowland dwellers who take to the mountains for recreation or sport, asthma should not prove a barrier provided it is well controlled – the same principles apply as for exercise-induced asthma in general. Some consideration should be given to the usability of some types of inhaler in low temperatures, and especially if also wearing thick gloves. Dry powder inhalers are more likely to work normally and be easier to use in these circumstances.

Depending on the nature of the climbing, mountaineering can be physically demanding, but skiing is likely to be accompanied by a higher level of aerobic exercise. The cold air and vigorous activity can prove a strong trigger for asthma and this might not be apparent until arriving on the slopes, which usually is far from the UK unless you ski in Scotland. A good self-management plan will include advice on what to do with your treatment should asthma symptoms get worse. A doubling up of the inhaled steroid is a common action to take when symptoms are not too bad but this may take a day or two to become effective. If previous experience showed this to be necessary then on your next skiing trip you might be best to increase your dose a few days before the holiday. While on the slopes simply wrapping a scarf around your face will warm the air you breathe in and reduce its tendency to cause bronchospasm. As with any holiday, it is essential to pack enough medication and not rely on getting supplies at your destination, which may prove impossible.

The best plan is to be prepared. A discussion with your asthma nurse or GP in advance might save you a lot of trouble when you are least able to get help.

Finally

None of the above is intended to discourage anyone with asthma to avoid exercise – quite the reverse. Asthma is not curable but it is highly treatable. With the right treatment you should be able to put it to the back of your mind and get on with the more important business of enjoying life.

Appendix A

References

General

- Global Initiative for Asthma. An international co-operation of asthma experts and organisations. The web site contains a wealth of useful information, the most detailed of which is the Global Strategy for Asthma Management and Prevention. Although a large file and intended mainly for health professionals it is well written in an understandable style and covers all aspects of asthma; http://www.ginasthma.com/workshop.pdf

- Cochrane Collaboration. The Cochrane Collaboration co-ordinates and publishes critical summaries of the medical literature. Their public site contains links to numerous health summaries of a variety of topics, including asthma; http://www.cochraneconsumer.com/index.asp?SHOW=Topics. See also: Cochrane Airways Group: http://www.cochrane.org/cochrane/revabstr/g150index.htm

- British Thoracic Society guidelines for the management of asthma (January 2003). Co-produced with the Scottish Intercollegiate Guidelines Network (SIGN). http://www.brit-thoracic.org.uk
- British Medical Journal: collected resources on asthma. Large archive of articles from previous issues of this main medical journal (written for health professionals); http://bmj.com/cgi/collection/asthma

Asthma in childhood

- International Study of Asthma and Allergies in Childhood (ISAAC), 'Worldwide variation in prevalence of symptoms of asthma, allergic rhinoconjunctivitis and atopic eczema' (Lancet, 1998; 351: 1225–1232); www.thelancet.com (use search archive to retrieve articles)

- Kaur, B., et al., 'Prevalence of asthma symptoms, diagnosis and treatment in 12–14 year old children across Great Britain (ISAAC UK)' (British Medical Journal, 1998; 316: 118–124); http://bmj.com/cgi/content/full/316/7125/118

- Oswald, H., et al., 'Outcome of childhood asthma in mid-adult life' (British Medical Journal, 1994; 309: 95–96); http://bmj.com/cgi/content/full/309/6947/95

- Anderson, H. R., et al., 'Trends in prevalence and severity of childhood asthma' (British Medical Journal, 1994; 308: 1600–1604); http://bmj.com/cgi/content/abstract/308/6944/1600

- The Childhood Asthma Management Program Research Group, 'Long-term effects of Budesonide or Nedocromil in Children with Asthma' (New England Journal of Medicine, 2000; 343: 1054–1063); http://content.nejm.org/cgi/content/full/343/15/1054

Allergy

- Shaheen, S., 'Discovering the causes of atopy' (British Medical Journal, 1997; 314: 98); http://bmj.com/cgi/content/full/314/7086/987

- Durham, S. R., et al., 'Long-term clinical efficacy of grass-pollen immunotherapy' (New England Journal of Medicine, 1999; 341: 468–475); http://content.nejm.org/cgi/content/full/341/7/468

- de Jong, M. H., et al., 'The effect of brief neonatal exposure to cows' milk on atopic symptoms up to age 5' (Archives of Disease in Childhood, 2002; 86: 365–369); http://adc.bmjjournals.com/cgi/content/abstract/archdischild%3b86/5/365

Pollution and environment

- Eisner, M. D., et al., 'Exposure to indoor combustion and adult asthma outcomes: environmental tobacco smoke, gas stoves, and wood smoke' (Thorax, 2002; 57: 973–978); http://thorax.bmj journals.com/cgi/content/abstract/57/11/973

- Grigg, J., 'The health effects of fossil fuel derived particles' (Archives of Disease in Childhood, 2002; 86: 79–83); http://adc.bmjjournals.com/cgi/content/abstract/archdischild%3b86/2/79

- Cook, D. G., and Strachan, D. P., 'Health effects of passive smoking: parental smoking and prevalence of respiratory symptoms and asthma in school age children' (Thorax, 1997; 52; 1081–1094); http://thorax.bmjjournals.com/cgi/content/abstract/52/12/1081

- Gilliland, F. D., et al., 'Effects of maternal smoking during pregnancy and environmental tobacco smoke on asthma and wheezing in children' (American Journal of Respiratory and Critical Care Medicine, 2001; 163: 2: 429–436); http://ajrccm.atsjournals.org/cgi/content/full/163/2/429

Self-management

- Lahdensuo, A., 'Guided self-management of asthma: how to do it' (British Medical Journal, 1999; 319: 759–760); http://bmj.com/cgi/content/full/319/7212/759

- Thoonen, B. P. A., et al., 'Self-management of asthma in general practice, asthma control and quality of life: a randomised controlled trial' (Thorax, 2003; 58: 30–36); http://thorax.bmjjournals.com/cgi/content/full/58/1/30

Complementary medicine

- Ernst, E., 'Complementary therapies for asthma: what patients use' (Journal of Asthma, 1998; 35: 667–671); http://www.ncbi.nlm.nih.gov/entrez/query.fcgi?cmd=Retrieve&db=PubMed&list_uids=9860087&dopt=Abstract

- Linde, K., et al., 'Acupuncture for the treatment of asthma' (The Cochrane Library); http://www.cochrane.org/cochrane/revabstr/ab000008.htm

- Linde, K., and Jobst, K. A., 'Homoeopathy for chronic asthma' (The Cochrane Library); http://www.cochrane.org/cochrane/revabstr/ab000353.htm

- Monteleone, C. A., and Sherman, A. R., 'Nutrition and asthma' (Archives of Internal Medicine, 1997; 157: 23–34); http://www.ncbi.nlm.nih.gov/entrez/query.fcgi?cmd=Retrieve&db=PubMed&list_uids=8996038&dopt=Abstract

- Berlowitz, D., et al., 'The Buteyko asthma breathing technique' (Medical Journal of Australia, 1995; 162: 53).

- Maher-Loughnan, G. P., et al., 'Controlled trial of hypnosis in the symptomatic treatment of asthma' (British Medical Journal, 1962; 2: 371–376).

- Ewer, T. C., and Stewart, D. E., 'Improvement in bronchial hyper-responsiveness in patients with moderate asthma after treatment with a hypnotic technique: a randomised controlled trial' (British Medical Journal, 1986; 293: 1129–1132).

- Balon, J., et al., 'A comparison of active and simulated chiropractic manipulation as adjunctive treatment for childhood asthma' (New England Journal of Medicine, 1998; 339: 1013–1020); http://content.nejm.org/cgi/content/full/339/15/1013

- Huntley, A., and Ernst, E., 'Herbal medicinal products for asthma: a systematic review' (Thorax, 2000; 55: 925–929); http://thorax.bmjjournals.com/cgi/content/full/55/11/925

- Huntley, A., et al., 'Relaxation therapies for asthma: a systematic review' (Thorax, 2002; 57: 127–131); http://thorax.bmjjournals.com/cgi/content/abstract/57/2/127

Appendix B

Drug Therapy: Class Examples

Only brief details of each drug are given here. Full details are included in the manufacturer's data sheets and can also be viewed within the medicines section of the NetDoctor website: http://www.netdoctor.co.uk/medicines/

The information is accurate at the time of writing but new information on medicines appears regularly. A health professional should always be consulted concerning the prescription and use of medicines.

Medicines and their possible side effects can affect individual people in different ways. The following lists some of the side effects that are known to be associated with these medicines. Side effects other than those listed may exist.

Steroids

Beclometasone inhaler

This medicine contains the active ingredient beclometasone dipropionate, which is a type of medicine known as a corticosteroid (or steroid). Corticosteroids are hormones produced naturally by the adrenal glands that have many important functions, including control of inflammatory responses.

Beclometasone is a synthetic corticosteroid and is used to decrease inflammation in the lungs. When inhaled into the lungs it is absorbed into the cells of the lungs and airways. Here it works by preventing the release of certain chemicals from the cells. These chemicals are important in the immune system and are normally involved in producing immune and allergic responses that result in inflammation. By decreasing the release of these chemicals in the lungs and airways, inflammation is reduced.

In asthma, the airways tighten due to inflammation and can also be blocked by mucus. This makes it difficult for air to get in and out of the lungs. By preventing the inflammation and excess mucus formation, beclometasone helps prevent asthma attacks. It is not used to treat an asthma attack.

Beclometasone is used via an inhaler device. This delivers the medicine directly into the lungs where it is needed. Used in this way, a smaller dose is required and the likelihood of side effects elsewhere in the body is reduced.

Warnings and advice

- Abrupt withdrawal of this medicine should be avoided.
- The mouth should be rinsed out with water after each dose of an inhaled corticosteroid, to prevent the development of oral thrush.
- Inhalers may cause an unexpected increase in wheezing (paradoxical bronchospasm) straight after using them. If this happens, stop using the inhaler immediately and consult your doctor. The medicine should be stopped and an alternative treatment found.
- Children on high dose long-term corticosteroid therapy should have their height monitored.

- This medicine should not be used to relieve an asthma attack as it will not work for this purpose. It must only be used as a regular medicine to prevent attacks. Make sure you carry your reliever (e.g. salbutamol inhaler) with you at all times to relieve attacks if they happen.
- When taken for long periods of time at high doses, corticosteroids have the potential to cause glaucoma, cataracts, thinning of the bones (osteoporosis), growth retardation in children and adolescents, and to decrease the functioning of the adrenal glands (glands that produce certain hormones). For this reason your doctor will prescribe the lowest effective dose for your symptoms, and monitor for these side effects.
- Blood potassium levels should be monitored in people with severe asthma, as low oxygen levels in the blood (hypoxia) and various asthma medicines, including this one, can lower blood potassium.
- Use with caution in active, inactive or dormant tuberculosis infection of the lungs.

Main common side effects
- yeast infection of the mouth (oral thrush)
- throat irritation
- allergic reactions such as skin rash, swelling of the lips, tongue and throat (angioedema) or narrowing of the airways (bronchospasm)
- cough and hoarseness.

How can this medicine affect other medicines?
There may be a decrease in the level of potassium in the blood when high doses of inhaled beclometasone are taken with the following:

- beta agonists, e.g. salbutamol, salmeterol, terbutaline
- theophylline
- diuretics, e.g. frusemide, bendrofluazide
- corticosteroids taken by mouth, e.g. prednisolone.

Other medicines containing the same active ingredients
AeroBec Autohaler, AeroBec Forte Autohaler, Asmabec Clickhaler, Asmabec Spacehaler, Beclazone inhaler, Beclazone Easi-Breathe, Becotide Inhaler, Becloforte inhaler, Becodisks, Becotide Rotacaps Filair Inhaler, Pulvinal Beclometasone Inhaler, Qvar Autohaler, Qvar Inhaler

Beta-2 agonists

Salbutamol

Salbutamol is a type of medicine known as a short-acting beta-2 agonist. It works by acting on receptors in the lungs called beta-2 receptors. Stimulation of these receptors causes the muscles in the airways to relax, allowing the airways to open.

Salbutamol is most commonly taken using an inhaler device. Inhaling the medicine allows it to act directly in the lungs where it is needed most. It also reduces the potential for side effects occurring in other parts of the body, as the amount absorbed into the blood through the lungs is lower than if it is taken by mouth.

Salbutamol when used as an inhaler is known as a 'reliever'. This is because it works very quickly to relieve asthma attacks or shortness of breath. Salbutamol inhalers can also be used to open the airways shortly before exercising.

Salbutamol tablets are sometimes prescribed if inhaled salbutamol is being used frequently to relieve shortness of breath. The tablets are taken regularly to help keep the airways open all the time and reduce the need for the inhaler.

Warnings and advice

- If this medicine fails to provide up to 3 hours' relief from shortness of breath, seek medical advice.
- Inhalers may (rarely) cause an unexpected increase in wheezing (paradoxical bronchospasm) straight after using them. If this happens, stop using the inhaler immediately and consult your doctor. The medicine should be stopped and an alternative treatment found.
- Blood potassium levels should be monitored in people with severe

asthma, as low oxygen levels in the blood (hypoxia) and various asthma medicines, including this one, can lower blood potassium.

Main side effects

- raised pulse rate
- awareness of the heart beat (palpitations)
- unexpected narrowing of the airways (paradoxical bronchospasm)
- low blood potassium level
- shaking, usually of the hands (tremor)
- anxiety and restlessness
- headache.

How can this medicine affect other medicines?

- This medicine should not be taken with beta-blockers, such as atenolol, propranolol or timolol. This is because beta-blockers have an opposite action to this medicine and cause the airways to narrow. This can result in breathing difficulties for people with asthma or chronic obstructive pulmonary disease.
- Salbutamol can potentially cause a serious decrease in the levels of potassium in the blood (hypokalaemia), which may result in adverse effects. This effect can be increased by the following medicines:
  - theophylline
  - corticosteroids, such as beclometasone and prednisolone
  - diuretics, such as bendrofluazide and frusemide
  - other beta-2 agonists, such as salmeterol.

Other medicines containing the same active ingredients

Aerolin Autohaler, Airomir Autohaler & Inhaler, Asmasal Clickhaler & Spacehaler, Asmaven Inhaler & Tablets, Maxivent Inhaler & Steripoules, Pulvinal Salbutamol Inhaler, Salamol products (Easi-Breathe, Inhaler, Steri-Neb ampoules), Salapin syrup, Salbulin Inhaler, Salbutamol Inhaler, Oral Solution & Tablets, Ventmax SR Capsules, Ventodisks, Ventolin products (Accuhaler, Inhaler, Evohaler, Nebules, Respirator Solution, Rotacaps, Syrup), Volmax Tablets

Sodium cromoglicate

Sodium cromoglicate is an anti-inflammatory medicine that is not a corticosteroid. It prevents tissues becoming inflamed when an allergic reaction occurs.

It is not fully understood how sodium cromoglicate prevents inflammation in asthma, but it is thought to work by preventing the release of inflammatory chemicals from cells called mast cells.

Mast cells are cells in the immune system that become sensitised in response to foreign particles, or allergens. When this happens, they release chemicals, including histamine, that go on to cause inflammation as part of the body's allergic response.

Allergic inflammation in the lungs is one of the causes of asthma. It causes mucus production and narrows the airways, making it difficult to breathe. As sodium cromoglicate reduces the inflammation in the lungs, it makes it easier to breathe and helps prevent asthma attacks. It should be used regularly, even when you have no asthmatic symptoms, to reduce the inflammation in the lungs. The medicine is taken using an inhaler device.

Warnings and advice

- This medicine should never be used to treat asthma attacks – you should keep your normal reliever inhaler, e.g. salbutamol or terbutaline, ready for this. Consult your doctor if you need to use your reliever more frequently than normal, or if it becomes less effective at treating attacks.

- If you have also been prescribed a reliever inhaler to open the airways when you are breathless (e.g. salbutamol or terbutaline), it is recommended that you use it before this preventive medicine. This opens the airways and allows the full dose of preventive medicine to be inhaled into the lungs.

- If it is necessary to stop treatment with this medicine, it should be withdrawn gradually over a period of one week, under supervision from your doctor. Symptoms of your asthma may recur. This medicine may very rarely make the airways narrow, causing shortness of breath (bronchospasm). If this happens, stop using it immediately and consult your doctor. The medicine should be stopped and an alternative treatment found.

Main side effects
- rash
- breathing difficulties due to a narrowing of the airways (bronchospasm)
- cough
- itchy rash (urticaria)
- throat irritation.

Other medicines containing the same active ingredients
Cromogen Inhaler, Easi-Breathe & Steri-Neb, Intal Inhaler, Nebuliser Solution & Spincaps

Leukotriene receptor antagonist

Montelukast
Montelukast is a type of medicine known as a leukotriene receptor antagonist. It works by blocking the action of leukotrienes, which are chemicals released by the body as part of the allergic and inflammatory response. Leukotrienes have effects in many areas of the body. In the lungs, they cause inflammation and increased mucus production in the airways. They also cause the muscles lining the airways to contract, which narrows the airways.

Montelukast should be taken regularly to prevent attacks, including when the asthma is under control. It is used for people whose asthma is not fully controlled with regular inhaled corticosteroids or short-acting beta agonist relievers such as salbutamol. It is also useful to prevent asthma caused by exercise. There are two brands of leukotriene receptor antagonist – montelukast ('Singulair' – suitable also for children – see below) and zafirlukast ('Accolate').

Warnings and advice
- If you take corticosteroids you should continue to take them while taking this medicine, even if your symptoms improve.

- This medicine should never be used to treat asthma attacks – you should keep your normal reliever inhaler, e.g. salbutamol or terbutaline, ready for this.
- Singulair 10mg is not recommended for children under 15 years of age, and Singulair Paediatric 5mg is not recommended for children under six years of age. Singulair Paediatric 4mg is not recommended for children under two years of age.
- In rare cases, people taking asthma medications may experience a rare condition known as Churg-Strauss syndrome. Consult your doctor if you experience any of the following while taking this medicine: flu-like symptoms, increasing breathlessness, pins and needles, numbness of the limbs or rash.
- This medicine should be taken at bedtime. Singulair Paediatric should be taken one hour before or two hours after food. Singulair for adults can be taken with or without food.
- People with an inherited disorder of protein metabolism (phenylketonuria) should be aware that Singulair paediatric chewable tablets contain aspartame, which is a source of phenylalanine.

Main side effects
- headache
- abdominal pain
- diarrhoea
- difficulty in sleeping
- thirst
- drowsiness
- nightmares
- skin rashes
- fever
- dizziness
- nausea and vomiting
- an extreme allergic reaction (anaphylaxis)
- cough
- irritability
- upper airway infections
- pain in the muscles and joints.

How can this medicine affect other medicines?
There are no significant interactions reported so far with montelukast; however, the manufacturer recommends that the following are used with caution, as they may decrease the blood level of montelukast:

- phenobarbitone
- phenytoin
- rifampicin.

Theophylline

Theophylline is a type of medicine called a xanthine bronchodilator. Theophylline causes the muscles surrounding the airways to relax, by a mechanism that is not fully understood. This allows the airways in the lungs to open.

Warnings and advice
- Some brands or preparations of medicine containing this active ingredient are not recommended for use in children under certain ages. Consult the package literature provided with the medicine for further information.
- Blood potassium levels should be monitored in people with severe airway obstruction, as low oxygen levels in the blood (hypoxia) and various airway medicines, including this one, can lower blood potassium.
- Smoking tobacco or cannabis, chewing tobacco or taking snuff can increase the removal of theophylline from the body, and increased doses of theophylline may be needed. Tell your doctor if you are giving up any of these, as your theophylline dose may need to be reduced.
- Different brands of sustained release theophylline are not interchangeable. You should make sure you know which brand you normally take, and that you receive the correct brand each time your prescription is dispensed.
- This medicine should not be taken with any other preparations containing theophylline or other xanthines.

Use with caution in:
- elderly people
- fever
- heart failure
- history of fits (seizures), e.g. epilepsy
- over-activity of the thyroid gland (hyperthyroidism)
- irregular heart beats (arrhythmias)
- liver disease
- peptic ulcers
- very high blood pressure (severe hypertension)
- viral infections.

Not to be used in:
- allergy to xanthines, e.g. aminophylline, theophylline, caffeine
- life-long inherited blood diseases which can cause a variety of symptoms, including mental health problems (porphyrias).

Main side effects
- headache
- restlessness
- fits (convulsions)
- low blood potassium level
- nausea and vomiting
- irritation to the lining or movements of the gut
- irritability
- increased heart rate (tachycardia)
- anxiety
- difficulty in sleeping
- awareness of the heart beat (heart palpitations).

How can this medicine affect other medicines?
- Children must not take ephedrine (present in many cough and cold remedies) while taking theophylline.
- The following medicines may *increase* theophylline blood levels:
  - aciclovir
  - allopurinol

- ○ calcium channel blockers, e.g. verapamil, nifedipine
- ○ methotrexate
- ○ isoniazid
- ○ flu vaccine
- ○ quinolone type antibiotics, e.g. ciprofloxacin, enoxacin, norfloxacin
- ○ macrolide type antibiotics, e.g. erythromycin, clarithromycin
- ○ cimetidine
- ○ oral contraceptives
- ○ disulfuram
- ○ fluvoxamine
- ○ interferons
- ○ mexiletine
- ○ oxpentifylline
- ○ tiabendazole
- ○ ticlopidine
- ○ propafenone
- ○ propranolol.

Your doctor may reduce your theophylline dose if you take any of these.

- The following medicines may *decrease* theophylline blood levels:
  - ○ aminoglutethimide
  - ○ barbiturates
  - ○ moracizine
  - ○ St John's wort
  - ○ sulphinpyrazone
  - ○ antiepileptic medicines, such as phenytoin, carbamazepine
  - ○ rifampicin
  - ○ rifabutin
  - ○ ritonavir.

Your doctor may increase your theophylline dose if you take any of these.

- Theophylline may decrease the blood levels of the following medicines, which may reduce their effects:
  - lithium
  - phenytoin
  - carbamazepine.

- Theophylline should not normally be taken with beta-blockers such as propranolol, as these oppose the effects of theophylline.
- There may be a risk of seizures if ketamine (an anaesthetic and pain-relieving drug which is also a drug of misuse) is taken with this medicine.
- There may be an increased risk of bleeding if this medicine is taken with lomustine (an anti-cancer drug).
- Theophylline may oppose the effects of the following medicines:
  - benzodiazepines, e.g. diazepam
  - adenosine (a drug used in treating heart rhythm problems).

The level of thyroid hormones in the body affects the way the body handles theophylline. If you have high thyroid hormone levels and start treatment to lower them, e.g. with medicines such as carbimazole, propylthiouracil or radioactive iodine, your doctor may need to decrease your theophylline dose. If you have low thyroid hormone levels and start treatment with thyroxine, your doctor may need to increase your theophylline dose.

Other medicines containing the same active ingredients
Nuelin, Nuelin SA, Slo-Phyllin, Uniphyllin Continus

Anticholinergic

Ipratropium
Ipratropium bromide is a type of medicine known as an antimuscarinic or anticholinergic bronchodilator. It is used to open the airways and assist breathing, in lung diseases such as asthma and bronchitis.

Ipratropium works by blocking receptors, called muscarinic receptors, that are found on the muscle surrounding the airways in the lungs. Stimulation of these receptors by a natural chemical called acetylcholine normally causes the muscle in the airways to contract, and this makes the airways narrow. Depending on how much the receptors are stimulated, this can cause difficulty in breathing. As ipratropium blocks the receptors, it stops the action of acetylcholine and allows the airways to open, making it easier to breathe.

Ipratropium is used regularly to keep the airways open in asthma and other conditions such as COPD. It does not work as quickly as the beta-agonist relievers. It is taken using an inhaler device.

Warnings and advice
- Inhalers may rarely cause an unexpected increase in wheezing (paradoxical bronchospasm) straight after using them. If this happens, stop using the inhaler immediately and consult your doctor. The medicine should be stopped and an alternative treatment found.
- Consult your doctor immediately if you experience sudden, rapidly worsening difficulty in breathing, or if this medicine becomes less effective than normal.
- Avoid contact of this medicine with the eyes, especially if you have, or are susceptible to, glaucoma. Seek medical advice if the medicine gets into the eyes.
- Consult your doctor immediately if you experience any of the following while using this medicine: eye pain or discomfort, blurred vision, visual haloes or coloured images in association with red eyes.

Use with caution in:
- closed angle glaucoma
- cystic fibrosis
- enlarged prostate gland (prostatic hypertrophy).

Not to be used in:
- allergy to ipratropium bromide or related medicines, e.g. atropine
- allergy to soya lecithin or related food products, e.g. soya beans or peanuts (applicable to Atrovent metered dose inhaler, Atrovent Autohaler and Atrovent Forte only).

Main side effects
- headache
- unexpected narrowing of the airways (paradoxical bronchospasm)
- nausea and vomiting
- cough
- throat irritation
- increased heart rate (tachycardia)
- dry mouth
- constipation
- difficulty in passing urine (urinary retention).

Other medicines containing the same active ingredients
Atrovent products (Aerocaps, Autohaler, Atrovent Forte, Inhaler & UDVs), Ipratropium Steri-Neb, Respontin Nebules

Useful Contacts

National Asthma Campaign

http://www.asthma.org.uk
The main UK charity specifically for asthma. Has a wide range of information available on-line and in printed form. Raises funds to support asthma research and offers independent help and advice.
   Helpline: 0845 701 0203

Allergy UK (formerly British Allergy Foundation)

http://www.allergyfoundation.com
Information, advice and support are available on most allergies, and chemical sensitivity, including details of the nearest allergy clinic. The website also lists manufacturers of products suitable for allergy sufferers.
   Helpline: 020 8303 8583

NHS – Giving Up Smoking

www.givingupsmoking.co.uk
Extensive information and help, including for ethnic communities, pregnancy, smoking in the workplace, e-mail based support and more. Locate your local NHS stop smoking service by entering your postcode in the custom search box.

NHS Smoking Helpline: 0800 169 0 169
Pregnancy Smoking Helpline: 0800 169 9 169

Quit

www.quit.org.uk
UK charity that helps smokers to quit. Quit has the longest established smoking helpline in the world and provides printed and telephone advice in multiple languages. Quit also has information to support teachers, lone parents, young people, people on low incomes and employers and runs training courses for health professionals.

Quitline (main number): 0800 00 22 00